Neuroscience

Information about Depressions, Phobias, and Tourette's

By Sally Stephens

Table of Contents

Chapter 1: Manic Depression

Manic anxiety is that state of anxiety in which the client suffers from state of mind swings which go between severe elation and anxiety. So while one minute the patient might feel on top of the world the other minute there will be emotions of anguish and vulnerability. Although there are lots of aspects that cause this type of depression genetic reasons are the most prominent ones. This means that two thirds of the people experiencing manic anxiety have somebody in their family also experiencing the exact same.

It is not only the state of minds of the person that get impacted by this but there are also physiological changes, there will be heightened activity at some time, insomnia at another and it also affects once social rhythms and thinking abilities.

Varying types of Manic Depression

Bipolar Anxiety
There are differing degrees of manic depression which means in some cases the ratio of an individual being depressed may be 3:1 while in other cases it could be as great as 37:1. What this means is that a person who has a provision of 3:1 will spend three times as much time depressed than elated. Scientists are also if the opinion that the condition of depression that the patients of Manic depression feel is rather more than that of typical depression and undoubtedly the chances of a person committing suicide is two times as much as somebody who is suffering from only anxiety or unipolar depression as it is called.

Combined Mania
Manic anxiety is also known to manifest itself in a combined state; this means that the people suffering from it will experience mania and depression at the exact same time. So they may experience agitation, stress and anxiety, fatigue, regret, impulsiveness, sleeping disorders, irritation, morbid and/or suicidal ideation, panic, fear, forced speech and rage all at the exact same time. A case in point would be somebody tearful or perhaps sobbing even when relatively appearing extremely cheerful or ecstatic. Such states are the most harmful and are prone to induce the optimum chances of substance abuse and even suicides.

Quick and ultradian cycles
Quick biking means that the individual tends to swing between one mood and the other rather often so while you might find them to be in an euphoric state at 10 in the early morning as if the world came from them you can see them at 11 and feel that they are the most powerless people in this world, although such type of our biking is not known to affect a ton of people there are fairly a great deal of cases who have greater cycles of a day or a month.

Signs of a Manic Depression

Manic depression is a mental illness that is also called manic depressive disorder. To some, it is known as bipolar affective disorder. Manic anxiety symptoms are known to be on the severe sides of the spectrum. They are either on the high-end or the low end. The high-end symptoms are understood to be the manic signs while the low end is known as the "hypo" signs or the depressive signs.

This kind of mental illness is tough to spot since the patient might appear to be going well after an episode of depression. Unknown to people around him, he becomes bright all of the abrupt not since he has overcome anxiety; it is just that he moved to mania, the other symptom of his illness.

The following are manic depression signs observed in patients who experience the manic or high-end of the psychological illness:

Severe generosity and euphoric mood.

Being inappropriate.

Inability to focus, always and easily sidetracked.

Talking extremely fast as a result of the racing ideas that flood the mind.

Extreme energy level, hyper activity and restlessness.

Excessive and uncharacteristic costs.

Incoherence and combined ideas.

Boost in sexual drive.

Intrusive conduct.

Overly aggressive conduct.

Very poor judgment

Thinking in his own extremely powers and impractical abilities.

Incredibly irritable.

Sleeps too little but still have way too much energy.

Abusive use of substances like cocaine, alcohol, and sleeping medications.

Falling into a rejection phase and not thinking that anything is very wrong with him.

The following manic depression signs are observed from clients on the low or depressed mode of the condition.

Unhappiness that remains for a significant length of time plant stress and anxiety and sensation of empty space.

A consistent sensation of tiredness and a really low energy level.

Feeling hopeless and always pessimistic.

Loss of sexual drive.

Failure to feel pleasure from anything.

Inability to focus.

A gnawing sense of regret and feeling worthless.

Lapse of memory.

Restlessness.

Severe irritation.

Inability to make logical choices.

Sleeping disorders or oversleeping.

A drastic loss or gain of cravings that causes either weight loss or gain.

Continuous body discomforts that cannot be validated by medical examinations.

Suicidal propensities.

Psychosis is another phenomenon that can be observed as a manic anxiety sign. It occurs in both manic and depressive modes of the disorder. It is characterized by hallucination and misconception that is often mistaken for schizophrenia (another form of mental disorder that also manifests hallucination and deception).

It is very important that proper diagnosis be done to tell whether it is manic depression sign or schizophrenia because the two types of mental disorder really need different kinds of mental and medical attention.

There are people who display combined manic-depressive signs. They manifest both the high and the low-end symptoms of the condition at the same time.

When to Look for Help
As discussed, it is challenging to determine if an individual has manic depressive condition. If you suspect that you or a liked one is struggling with this mental disorder, it would be best if you drop in a psychiatrist to totally assess your condition instantly since the person with this illness has a very unpredictable and unsteady conduct. It can go from shoplifting to promiscuous sexual behavior to suicide. What's more, these habits might appear within a short time period.

Proper diagnosis of the manic depressive signs is essential to provide the appropriate treatment needed by the client. The symptoms are puzzling. The assistance of expert people is very important to recuperate effectively. Administration of medication is generally needed to stabilize the patient. Medications would help a patient react well to other forms of psychiatric treatments just like psychotherapy and cognitive treatment.

Some Qualities

Manic depression is also commonly known as bipolar disease. It involves rotating mood swings that range from a high point called mania, down to a low point referred to as anxiety. The reason that it is also referred to as bipolar illness is because of the state of mind swings from the high pole to the low pole. Sometimes an individual with bipolar disease will experience remarkable switches in their mood extremely quickly.

It is more common that an individual will manic depression will experience these state of mind swings in a gradual way. Among the problems that people with this disease have to contend with is that this disease can affect their capability to believe clearly; also it can impact their judgment. A more serious affect is when their social conduct is modified by bipolar disease. It can cause humiliating and serious problems in a social setting. Manic anxiety is a chronic condition that is repeating, but with proper treatment, it can be a workable illness.

Some attributes of the more extreme episodes that an individual with manic anxiety may experience are psychotic signs. Some of the more typical of these signs consist of hallucinations, like hearing things or seeing things that are actually not there. Another extreme characteristic of a person with this disease is deceptions. Delusions can trigger an individual with bipolar disease to actually believe in certain things that normal sensible thinking would otherwise not really believe in. Psychotic symptoms may include that person believing that someone has unique hero like powers, or someone is a president or king from another spot.

Typically, these kinds of signs happen throughout the peak of their state of mind swing. Some characteristics of a person that has bipolar disease can also involve a delusion of worthlessness, regret or thinking that somebody is in terrible trouble. These signs generally happen during the low point in their state of mind swing. Not all qualities are serious. In fact, most attributes can include irritation, trouble sleeping and not having the ability to sit still. On the depression side of milder characteristics of manic depression can include not wanting to mingle, not wanting to talk and feeling sad and blue.

Manic anxiety does have some qualities that are nothing more than a misconception. Many people believe that an individual cannot have a normal life with it or that they cannot get better. The truth is that many people that have bipolar illness have an effective profession and a happy family. Another myth is that manic anxiety only affects their mood. It can also impact their sleeping habits, capability to concentrate, energy and appetite. While medicine is a well-known treatment for manic anxiety, there are self assistance things that can be done. Manic depression signs can be managed by regular exercise, lots of sleep and eating right, just to name a few. Dealing with bipolar disease can be challenging. With the right treatment, coping abilities and an outstanding support system, a person with manic depression can lead a typical and happy life.

What Can Cause a Manic Depression?

A manic anxiety is different from a normal depression in the simple fact that an individual not only has periods where he feels extremely sad, he also has amount of times where he feels himself perfectly well. Although this may sound good, this is not the case as people loose reality of who they are and what they can do. Some people for example believe they are superman or god and will act in the exact same way.

There are tons of possible causes that are the root of this order but the truth is we do not know exactly how a condition like Manic Depression is caused. However, from what we do know scientific research has revealed that there is a hereditary link. The occurrence of this condition is higher among clients where their father or mother also had manic anxiety. This doesn't clarify the whole process why some people do and others will not get this condition.

The limit theory says that everybody has a chance on manic anxiety, but for a single person the chance is much higher than for the other. If you will get a specific condition like manic depression would depend on the amount of demanding life events. So this theory specifies that it is a mix between level of sensitivity and demanding life events.

Although this idea has some extremely strong points, it also has some defects as it is a really general one not indicating the extremely complex structure of the brain.

Many ladies who have been diagnosed with Manic Depression sometimes long to have kids, but often really wonder what the chances are that they will pass it onto their children. They know all too well the impacts of the disorder and wish to not pass it on to another generation. Studies have shown that manic depression is usually found in the genes, and is given the bloodline. That statement does not always mean you will pass it on, it means there is a good chance.

If manic depression (also referred to as Bipolar Disorder) is found relatively typically in your family history, your chances increase. People who have no history found in their genealogy have virtually no threat, less than 1%. If you have bipolar illness, the approximate chances of you passing it to your kid is 5-15%.

Approximately twenty five percent of adult bipolar patients report having their first manic episode right before they were twenty years of age. There have been research studies that have reported kids as young as 5 years of age showing indications of small manic episodes. There is a lot of research being carried out on manic anxiety. There are institutions reporting that they will quickly be able to do a screening to identify if you do in fact carry the gene that might pass it on to your children.

If you actually believe your kid might have bipolar affective disorder, a calm and nurturing environment can reduce the chances of your kid having major manic episodes. This is a condition that sometimes needs a trigger to so as to become progressive. A violent or demanding environment can cause trigger manic depression, and trigger episodes to increase and become more severe. Be sure to stay in constant contact with your doctor to remain on top of the most recent Bipolar Medications and treatment options available.

For a long time, it's been well recognized among bipolar scientists that mania and anxiety can affect sleep patterns. When a bipolar patient is experiencing severe mania, he might be too manic to sleep. On the other hand, when he is going through a depressive episode, he might sleep too much and actually not feel like rising.

What lots of researchers have discovered as well is that the manic/depressive cycle works both methods. To put it simply, a lack of sleep can potentially activate manic episodes. Research studies are demonstrating that approximately 60 percent of bipolar suffers who have gone through a manic attack experience some sort of interruption in their regular sleep cycle previous to having the attack.

We all have had experiences when at the most troublesome time possible, we were interrupted by life. Social rhythm disruptions, or SRDs, are life events that interrupt our recognized regimens like a sleep pattern. In regular people, i.e., those not suffering from bipolar affective disorder, this is not a huge offer. We shrug it off and ultimately go back to our routine patterns. In bipolar clients, though, social rhythm disruptions in their sleep pattern can straight set off a manic attack.

This is why tons of healthcare experts advise that their bipolar patients write up a sleep schedule for themselves and keep to it. This means going to sleep at the same time each night and getting up at the same time each early morning - even on weekends. Keeping to this schedule will keep "social rhythm disruptions" to a minimum and lessen the risk of a manic attack. As a basic rule, following a sleep schedule also means not resting when you have had a hard time sleeping the previous night. Sleeping would simple be another form of social rhythm interruption and would not help in the long term.

Absence of sufficient sleep will make anyone irritable and grouchy. Most of us, though, will just be able to fall asleep the next night and "catch up on our sleep" and be perfectly great the next day. Bipolar people cannot always do this. They might be unable to go to sleep thus setting off a manic attack the next morning. The manic attack will minimize their desire to sleep and they will not sleep much the next night either. It is a discouraging and possibly deadly cycle.

It can be hard for a bipolar person to keep to a sleep schedule without the help of members of the family. Consisting of family members in the treatment discussions with the health care provider benefits everybody. It helps the family members to understand how seriously essential it is that the bipolar patient keeps to a routine sleeping regimen. It helps the bipolar person by giving him psychological assistance and making him feel less abnormal.

Strong family support is specifically important when the bipolar victim is a teen who, in many cases, is already going through a stressful duration in his life at a time when peer pressure tends to make castaways of those that don't appear to be normal. But even in adult cases of bipolar disease, the assistance of a caring family cannot be over estimated.

Some Truths

Manic anxiety is a kind of mental disorder that is commonly described as bipolar illness. This can be recognized by the person's low and high mood swings which can shift at anytime and for any reason. It can impact the person's state of mind along with their energy and how they work throughout their daily lives.

This certain kind of anxiety can affect both males and females and can manifest itself at any age. However, it more typically starts when the person is a teen or young person. Many health experts believe that this condition can be passed along through the hereditary code in people and can affect someone no matter what race or ethnic group they come from.

People with this issue can injure not only themselves - but also the people that are around them. There are medications that they can take - which will help to control the symptoms and the mood changes. among the best ways to control the issue is to understand that things that can set you off.

Normally there is a pattern that can trigger an episode and understanding what it is and how to avoid it will help. Besides being treated regularly you must make certain that you get the proper amount of sleep. Basically anything that can impact your mood in an unfavorable or excessively positive way can send you into an episode.

Many people think that when you have manic anxiety you will be sad or angry all the time by different life events or even daily things. Nevertheless, it can also impact how happy and fired up you are. One 2nd you can be so thrilled about something that you are acting oddly and the next 2nd you could be exceptionally sad or mad about something else.

What Changes in the Brain?

With contemporary brain imaging, it ends up being clear that bipolar is not a disorder, but a brain disease, as real as cancer or a cold. While science is still examining the distinctions between the brain of a typical person and the brain of a bipolar person; here are four distinctions between the two.

1.) Ventral Striatum
The forward striatum permits the brain to procedure benefits, just like rejoicing after eating or making love. If somebody suffers from bipolar, this part will be overactive and have a 30% loss in the amount of noodle.

The forward striatum also aids in judgment, just like what is thought about typical or moral. Since bipolar persons suffer a reduction in this part of the brain, they will be susceptible to overspending or sexual indiscrimination, especially when manic.

2.) Prefrontal Cortex
The prefrontal cortex enables the brain to process and guideline feeling, an important part of impulse control. For example, when one feels upset, they don't head out and hit the very first person they see.

In those with bipolar disorder, there is a 20% to 40% decrease in gray matter material in the prefrontal cortex, triggering rash behavior and anger control issues.

3.) Amygdala
The amygdala manages facial expressions and tones of voice. For example, if you see a person you like on the technique, neural transmittals will occur in your brain, telling you to smile. In the bipolar brain, there is a loss of gray matter in this location, causing a hold-up response in facial expressions.

4.) Hippocampus
In those with bipolar disorder, the hippocampus has lost branches that connect nerve cells, causing a loss of a capability to discriminate between threat and benefit, triggering a state of stress and anxiety.

When to Look for Help

When you are manic, you are impatient and hostile towards others since they just can't seem to 'see' what you are talking about, and they never can. As a result, you could wind up annoyed with them and start to harm even those that you care about, physically injuring your children or partner.

Also, when you are manic you have an inflated ego and sense of self-esteem that usually comes with delusions of grandeur, and a self-esteem that triggers you to really believe you have more wit, guts, creativity, and artistry than everyone else.

When you are manic, you aren't yourself, and you aren't a very good person to be around. You are energized with racing ideas that are never on the same topic for enough time, so that you sleep that much less. Alcohol and substance abuse is common, with other kinds of self-destructive behavior like obnoxious and combative conduct.

Is that all? Obviously not. Here's the absolute worst part - you are like this only half of the time. The other half you are depressed enough to want to kill yourself. It does not take a great deal of believing to know why they call this the "fine insanity". It's as you really seethe when you are struggling with such an illness; and like regular insanity, you truly don't know that you are mad. That is what is so miserable about the manic-depressive health problem. The symptoms displayed can result in damaging activities.

When you see any of such indications, do not waste time at all. Talk to your doctor instantly, so that you can get help before you do something extreme to yourself or your really loved ones.

Tests in Teenagers

Manic anxiety is a bipolar or mental condition issue that is not only discovered in teens but in every individual. It has to do with how people feel at every time toward something, themselves, and even to people around them.

As a teen, have you ever experienced a state of mind swing circumstances where your mood changes from one direction to the other? For instance you are incredibly happy now and then some hours later you are incredibly miserable for no great reason?

If that holds true then you are having manic depression and it is a mental illness issue. Or let's say you feel you are the best in what you do amongst your mates then all of a sudden; you started feeling you are not good enough to compete at any given level.

It is very crucial to keep in mind that it is not all the time that you experience these emotions that you are struggling with bipolar affective disorder. Everyone has had some dreadful experiences and in most cases; having a reflection on such experiences can make you feel bad sometimes.

Sure when it happens like this; then you aren't struggling with any form of disorder as such feeling is for the time being and will go as time progresses. But on the other hand; when you are experiencing such some feeling routinely and on a frequent basis then there is the problem of anxiety and it is finest advised to see a doctor closest to you.

Manic anxiety tests in teens does not have any format neither does it follow the conventional ways of carrying out diagnosis on a client like blood tests, x-ray and the rest. It needs rather some questions that the clients really need to ask themselves and supply answers to such.

Here are some of the bipolar disorder tests in teens:

How is your social life?
Your social life as a teen should be great and impeccable in regards to mixing up with your mates and people around you as a teenager. If you do not see any reason to blend with them and this happens all the time, then it is possible that you are having this condition issue.

Are you happy with yourself and those around you?
Manic anxiety can come in this form especially when you do not always rejoice with either your members of the family or friends. Hence, you blame them for the problems and miseries you are having in life.

Are you quickly provoked?
If you are the type of person that gets quickly inflamed at the sight of something or people around you like your friends then you should try as much as you can to see
your doctor for therapy especially to prevent this disorder issue from hitting its innovative phase as people suffering from this psychological imbalance tend to unnecessarily get inflamed.

Do you go to spots like club to look for happiness all the time?
It is really true that you can go to some places like a club to pass time and have some type of fun but you cannot go there to look for joy and even if you do; it
cannot be all the time. Such joy will not stand the test of time and there is need for you to identify the root of this problem before it eats you up.

A lot of teenagers nowadays even seek the companion of alcohol and drugs to stay happy and comfortable. This has to stop as you will only ruin your life in addition to health in the long run.

You need to identify these manic depression tests in your life as a teenager well to ensure that you are on the right road to living a typical life just as your mates are doing.

Talking about carrying out tests ...
Do you know that although you can use the above tests to determine manic anxiety in your life as a teenager there is a mistake you will not want to make? This mistake will be so devastating that it can make your condition problems to reach a deteriorating phase. Discover how you can stay away from these errors.

How to Decrease the Signs

It's a tested fact that a manic depressive person could be crippled by the irregularity of his/her state of minds. This psychological health condition would be exceptionally distressing not only to the patient but to other close family members and friends as well. The great news is that there are some things that you can do to decrease the impacts and symptoms of what can be a sometimes disabling condition. By learning to organize your manic depressive state, you can reduce having the bipolar label positioned upon you.

First, you will want to learn as much as you potentially can about your mindset. The more realities that you recognize about being a manic depressive, the better are your chances in keeping the symptoms at bay and potentially eliminating the condition from affecting your daily life. After all, the supreme goal is to live manic depressive symptom completely free.

Second, you will want to remove stress whenever possible. It is very essential that you avoid having a demanding state as your state of mind swings are intimately connected to your level of tension. You should try to always manage your difficult situations as best as you can with the least amount of excitement. It can be very helpful to enroll in meditative workouts just like yoga and Pilates. Many individuals report that this has worked wonders for controlling their bipolar disorder.

Next, make sure to engage in a routine exercise program. Not only will this rejuvenate your body but it has been proven to work wonders for your mind. A regular walking regimen is great for starters; From there you can develop to whatever you are comfortable with. In really short time, you will be astonished at how a regular workout can be beneficial for your mental state in addition to your physical state.

Next, you want to capture a full night's rest as usually as you can. Avoid activities that hinder a very good night's sleep. The suggestion is 7 to 8 hours of nightly sleep. Upon awakening, try not to skip breakfast. This is a very crucial meal to get your day off to a really good start. Mentioning meals be certain to have great eating habits and stay away from the scrap.

Finally, you should know when to get support from others. Keep in mind that this is not a battle that you ought to combat alone. Throughout history, there have been lots of popular people that have been detected as bipolar. Those that have looked for the aid of experts have gone on to lead rather normal lives. Following the advice of professionals will enable you to keep control over your manic depressive episodes and live a fuller life.

Coping with Losses and trauma

Dealing with loss of family can be specifically difficult for those who struggle with manic depression. Not only are they trying to cope with the traumatic experience, but they are also attempting to stay stable and attempting to keep away from a depressive or manic episode as a result of the stress it triggered. Some with manic anxiety may even need to seek extra support to handle the grief or anxiety that the terrible event causes.

Everybody deals with sorrow or anxiety in a different way during a loss or trauma. Coping with manic anxiety can be a delicate balancing act. If something creates a lot of stress or stress and anxiety for them, they can easily become overloaded and slip into mania or depression. When grieving, it is not unusual for someone to feel depressed. Nevertheless, if somebody with manic depression grieves and feels depressed, they need to make a mindful effort to try to avoid having a full-blown depressive episode. However in some cases, the looming depressive episode just cannot be kept away from.

A support system is absolutely necessary when handling trauma. Family, friends, support system, and psychological health specialists can all help the manic anxiety person through the terrible event. Typically, all it takes is an understanding individual to listen to the person with manic anxiety and offer motivation.

Helping relieve some of the stress and duties from the person suffering from manic anxiety can help them concentrate on maintaining balance and handling the extra stress the trauma has triggered. Motivate the manic depression person to take some time for himself to do something they take pleasure in. Taking a walk with the person can help offer workout and social stimulation, which is usually not having. Lots of people with manic anxiety tend to separate themselves when under too much tension. This can be detrimental to their health and emotional well-being.

If the person with manic depression begins to experience nightmares, sleeplessness, stress and anxiety, restlessness, distress, or if they are repeatedly remembering or reliving the acts of the distressing event, they probably need extra support from their psychiatrist or doctor in order to handle the trauma. Medication can help the person to manage the anxiety and distress triggered by the event. It is better to get the additional help essential to control the effects of the trauma and avoid an episode than to neglect getting aid and deal with the anxiety and distress plus a manic or depressive episode.

People with manic depression who have experienced trauma or a loss should think about broadening their support group to include assistance particularly associated to the trauma. Depending on the nature of the trauma, support system and specialized counseling might be available. If the person with manic depression had not been getting therapy, they should think about doing so to help them through this difficult time.

How to Treat Manic Depression

What is manic depression and how can it be treated? Manic depression is also generally called bipolar disorder. To explain it, it usually appears with a ton of either highs or lows in one's conduct as well as feelings. This is identified by gradual significant state of mind switches that normally affect a person's judgment in addition to social behavior. As this condition impacts one's ideas, it definitely triggers shame together with other serious troubles.

An individual with manic depression might in some cases feel so active and might even like to be actually efficient. They may often actually feel great about themselves, and it can even reach a point that they would believe that they actually are a lot better than other individuals around them. But also often they can truly feel ineffective, that their efforts are useless both in their individual and expert lives, and more than these, they also may have self-destructive propensities. So to sum everything up, manic depression is characterized by mood instability which can actually be critical and can prevent a patient from living a typical life.

Typically, manic disorder often is not truly identified. And it is really true that even if a person is detected with it, in some cases the chances for them to get a real great treatment are extremely restricted. One reason is since the reason for this disorder is brought about by a ton of factors that all act up together. So detects actually needs to done at an early stage of the condition before it really disengages the patient from a regular environment. It can also be a result of problems in brain functions that might not support them as they process life events making them anxious and stressed. So what can actually be the best manic depression treatment?

Manic anxiety treatment is long-lasting. It consists of both medication and psychosocial treatments. Medications or "mood stabilizers" include lithium treatment that helps manage the reoccurrence of manic and depressive episodes. Another medication is carbamazepine which is an anticonvulsant, to help stabilize a person in the most hard bipolar episode. Treatments also can consist of antipsychotic medications just like Quetiapine, Olanzapine and Chlorpromazine. Some also use antidepressants, though the efficiency of antidepressants are yet to be debated on.

Actually manic anxiety treatment will not treat the condition. Treatment is done to help the patient manage the bipolar episodes they experience. Psychosocial treatments, which include talk psychotherapy, are used to educate, guide and support a patient and his family. Although a client can voluntarily admit himself for hospitalization, particularly during their manic episodes, these psychosocial interventions are shown more efficient to increase an individual's mood stability, and can even help them enhance their functions. A treatment that integrates medication and psychosocial treatment is essential in dealing with the disorder. Even during treatments, bipolar episodes will still occur but with continuous treatment and with close coordination with a doctor, a full-blown episode can be stopped.

Alternative Treatment Approaches

The Following are Alternative Manic Depression Treatments:

Organic Treatment
Herbs and mood-stabilizing compounds can also be used in Bipolar affective disorder treatment. Herbs are compounds not essentially needed by the body. Nonetheless, research studies show that herbs can curb the signs of state of mind conditions. This is credited to the medicinal actions and properties that they have. Basil, Black root, Bog myrtle, Borage, Ceanothus, Chamomile, Chervil, Damiana, Ginseng, Heather, Girl's slipper, Lemon balm, Mugwort, Nettle, Oats, Pimpernel, Primrose, Night, Saffron, Sage, Sedge root, St. John's wort, Thistle, holy or blessed, Valerian, and American are examples of herbs that are believed to be able to avert psychological conditions.

Phototherapy
Seasonal depression, or more commonly known as seasonal anxiety, is primarily attributed to the absence of sunshine throughout winter. Supplemental artificial light effectively deals with the condition by exposing the patient 30 minutes a day in front of unique bright-light equipment. This is effective in raising the spirits of about sixty percent to eighty percent of those affected by seasonal winter season anxiety.

Acupuncture
Quite a few research studies have revealed that acupuncture treatment might work in the recovery of manic anxiety disorder. A medical/scientific analysis would be that the acupuncture points rouse the central nervous system, thereby encouraging the release of beneficial chemicals into the muscles, spine, and brain. This would eventually promote the body's natural healing capabilities. Research has shown that acupuncture treatment might customize brain chemistry by changing the discharge of neurotransmitters and neurohormones in a positive way.

Aromatherapy
Aromatherapy treatment has been observed to help in the milder types of anxiety. It could ease mental fatigue and helps in giving better sleep. Nevertheless, it is a good idea that an extremely depressed individual gets further support and treatment. The impact of Aromatherapy is more effective when it is used as a complimentary therapy by supplementing other therapies. Vital oils utilized for Aromatherapy depression treatment are basil, bergamot, cedar wood, clary sage, frankincense, grapefruit, geranium, lavender, lemon, jasmine, myrrh, neroli, rose, sandalwood, spruce, orange and ylang.

Massage Treatment
Massage is mainly employed to improve blood flow in muscles, alleviate stress and muscle spasms, and help the lymphatic and nerve systems. The results of better blood circulation lead to the decline of the negative consequences of anxiety, tension and depression. Massage has also been understood to change patients' brain patterns and use useful aid for patients

suffering from stress and anxiety and depression. This is primarily as a result of the enjoyable experiences that massage provides to the body.

Music Treatment
Research shows that the electromagnetic field that surrounds our head attunes to the electro-magnetic field of the world earth when we are in a condition of deep relaxation or reflection. Listening to calming music as a result makes the majority of people loosen up and this treatment is believed to work wonders in people struggling with manic anxiety.

Meditation
Research studies have suggested that during meditation, the body attains a condition of extensive rest. Together, the brain and mind happen to become more alert, hence showing a condition of peaceful awareness. In current times, meditation treatment has turned into an increasingly important tool for finding a tranquil sanctuary of leisure and stress relief in cases of manic anxiety.

Using a Support System

Having actually identified with bipolar disorder can be one of the most demanding and hard experiences of an individual's life. To learn to manage bipolar affective disorder better, whether yourself, with friend or families, it is necessary to build and keep a strong support group.

A support group is a group of people who come together to offer unconditional psychological assistance to the person with bipolar illness, these people need to have the desire to comprehend the struggle and problems of dealing with bipolar affective disorder. They can consist of families, good friends, support system, therapists, psychological health caseworkers, and even physicians.

Having family and closed friends who use psychological support is an exemptionally valuable property to those struggling with bipolar affective disorder. In times of situation, when people impacted by the condition feel overwhelmed by suicidal ideas or feel that their life is spiraling out of control, they really need to know who they can depend on for aid and comfort. This is where the support system is so essential.

A manic anxiety support group is an outstanding source of peer support. Support system can help lots of people deal with the emotional elements by offering a safe spot to share experiences and learn from other ones who are dealing with comparable situations. Within a support system for bipolar disorder, there are likely to be people who have experienced the ups and downs of bipolar illness and who is the best person to share their experience but them.

An individual with a manic depressive health problem may feel isolated and separated in the disorder. They may also feel alone in their struggle to manage the signs. Attending a support system can show the person that they are not alone in their journey to healing from bipolar illness.

Support groups for bipolar affective disorder are usually not specifically for bipolar disorder, and generally developed for those who have any mood disorders, including bipolar illness and clinical depression. If you need more information about such support group, your therapist or psychiatrist should be able to give some guidance on some of the regional support groups that are available.

When signing up with a support system, somebody with bipolar disorder should try to participate in whether they are in situation or doing well. If somebody new goes to the group and only sees other ones who are in dilemma, it may give the beginner a sense of anguish and despondence. The idea is to support one another through the journey of recovery. Throughout a regular duration between episodes, someone can be a light of want to members who are having difficulty handling the condition.

In the current age of innovation, one can find many Web support groups and chat rooms developed as manic depression support system. These can be a pretty good resource for those who experience the disorder. Nevertheless, being active in Web support system is not enough and should not replace the going to of local support groups. This is because somebody with bipolar disorder can have a disposition to isolate himself. Attending a regional support system supplies positive social interactions with people who comprehend the difficulty that the manic depressive person is facing and help stop him from isolating from society.

How to Feel Happy again

Generally, bipolar affective disorders, can be put under the general category of anxiety, but its manifestations are very different as compared to the other ones. A bipolar affective disorder is identified by 2 relatively complete opposite habits that are found in one person. This condition has no recognized remedy, but through treatment, the symptoms may be manageable. Like medical conditions just like diabetes or cardiovascular disease, bipolar illness needs to be kept under control for the rest of a person's life.
This condition is really intricate, hence making it challenging for specialists to detect. Many people have had to deal with the condition for some years right before they seek a diagnosis and a corresponding treatment. Specialists really believe it is brought on by an imbalance in the brain chemistry, but some research studies are showing that there may be a hereditary element. The illness itself might take place intermittently throughout a person's life.

Bipolar affective disorders are primarily dealt with by medication. A combination of anti-psychotics, mood stabilizers, anti-convulsants, and antidepressants are generally administered to clients to manage the severe state of mind swings of the condition. Throughout treatment, an individual may expect to have his/her medication change all throughout its course. A single proposed dosage does not always have the exact same impact at all times. Some cases call for the application of psychotherapy, but this method experiences limited success if done without medication.

Bipolar affective disorders can become really hazardous when without treatment. Around seventeen percent of unattended bipolar disorder clients commit suicide. For those who experience major anxiety, the rate of suicide is only about 10 percent.

Dealing with manic anxiety can be a genuine challenge for the individual suffering with the illness. It is hard for the person experiencing it, and on those around them. Understanding that your condition has serious results upon those you love can even serve to intensify the conditions. Knowing what to expect from your health problem and planning out approaches of handling the signs goes a long way in minimizing the stress and stress and anxiety of this serious health problem.

Step One: Know that it is a disease. Manic depression is not a personal shortage. It is not something you choose to have. You aren't sympathizing with yourself. You aren't over-acting. You have a real health problem. Do not let what other ones might believe influence how you feel about yourself, and treat yourself. The majority of what those who have not dealt with mental illness know about the realities have plenty of false information. While you might not be able to educate everyone, focus on handling those closest to you as they discover what bi-polar illness is, and how to successfully help you deal with the health problem.

Step 2: learn to keep tension to a minimum. Tension is a big factor in triggering manic depressive attacks. You may feel like your body has betrayed you after being detected with manic depression. Do not enable the emotions of betrayal to overwhelm you. It is alright to feel upset about the simple fact that your world has been turned upside down. That's natural for anyone. Recognize the need for anger and sorrow and let them have their spot, but do not concentrate on them. Instead, focus on all of the positive things that you can do to make your life fuller and happier. Knowing what the problem is can be half the battle.

Step 3: Keep precise track of your medications. Your recommended medications will help you manage the hold that manic anxiety has on your life. In order to be able to live your life to the maximum you really need to have those psychological low and high under complete control. Your medicines are your lifeline. Make a chart with what medications to take when on it, and follow it religiously.

Step Four: Keep a strategy. Just like your medicine chart, a plan of action for day-to-day needs is a great way to be sure you do not misplace the things you need to do. Make substantial to do lists and follow them. Set each item on the list as a little objective. If there are larger products that need to be accomplished break them up into tinier individual objectives to get there. That will keep you from feeling too overwhelmed by large tasks. Completing each product will give you a sense of achievement, and settling your day will make you feel terrific and independent.

Step 5: Keep a diary. Speaking about your issues to loved ones is a great way to alleviate the emotions of loneliness and tension of a mental disorder. Another essential way to deal with your disease is to keep a journal. Write in it every day. The great and the bad. That way when you are feeling actually upset, or psychological, you can look back and see what made you feel that way right before and how you handled it, or what made you happy on good days and how you can get out of the bad regions this time.

Keeping a journal can also help to show you if you are making enhancements and the bad days are less than the good ones. It can also signal you to trouble if the bad days are beginning to catch up to the good ones in number. Many of all, keeping a journal just helps in allowing you to talk it out with yourself.

You can live a terrific, happy, and productive live while dealing with bi-polar condition. Your good friends and your family will be with you on your journey and you can be independent and delight in the world again with just a little planning.

Caring for People with a Manic Depression

Every day in your life, you experience things that may either give you a happy or a sad feeling. Stressors are always present in the environment and within you. It is the ability of the body to manage it that makes you adapt to the norms. There are circumstances that the feeling of happiness is distorted to a frenzied feeling. On the other hand, the feeling of sadness can be altered to a depressive state. These situations happen when you are experiencing a bipolar affective disorder. This disorder doesn't only manifest manic episodes but depressive episodes too.

There are two episodes of this disorder as pointed out above. The manic episode is characterized by verbosity, ostentation, sleeplessness, flight of ideas (shifting from one subject to another), hypersexuality, distractibility, social intrusiveness, and psychomotor agitation. While the depressive episode can be manifested by tiredness, emotions of worthlessness, somatic grievances, lessened hygiene, failure to make choices, social withdrawal, and suicidal ideations. The episodes can last for hours, days, weeks, or perhaps months. The 2 can interchangeably happen, but the period of their incident will depend upon the type of bipolar illness the person has.

The first top priority for this kind of person is security. As you can observe, security is usually the priority when you handle people who have mental disorders. This is since they do not have the capability to figure out things. When the person has a depressive condition, it is incredibly essential to evaluate for the presence of any suicidal ideation. If the ideation is evident in the person, then you'll have to make sure that the environment is safe. Get rid of all sharp things, bottles, ropes, or any products which he can use to harm himself. Have an individual supervise him for 24 hours to monitor his actions.

You should also offer rest during this episode to make up for the fatigue he is experiencing. On the other hand, when the person has moved into a manic episode, you should be additional watchful because he has now sufficient energy to execute his suicide strategy. The person can be hyperactive so there is a greater danger for that person to injure himself. Offer him with varied activities that can channel his energy, such as duping newspapers, and you also need to set the limits for them.

The next primary concern would be nutrition. This can be an important element of their care because both disorders include existing problems handling food. Manic individuals have hyperactivity, and they hardly pay more attention to food because their attention is concentrated on other unimportant things. Since most of the time they are in movement, you can provide high-calorie finger foods like French fries and sandwiches. It will renew the energy they've been using and also please their needs temporarily. For a person who has depressive episodes, you may really need patience to be able to persuade him to eat. Give him time to finish his meal since they even lack energy to eat.

The most important and gentle elements in caring for these types of people are empathy and persistence. For manic individuals, you can represent the role of a father who protects and controls their unsuitable habits. When it comes to the depressive ones, you can depict a mother figure that can be available to listen to them. You have to always be there for them. Assist them to accomplish their optimum level of health where they can be a practical member of society.

What Are Phobias?

A real phobia is a severe form of fear or stress and anxiety activated by a particular
Circumstances (such as going outside) or item (such as spiders), even when There is no risk.

Phobia is basically just an irrational fear of something. In today's society it is easy to find at least
one phobia for every single person you encounter. What triggers phobias though is still an often
pondered question.

Phobias should not be puzzled with easy worries, like being afraid of a lion as that is a normal
protective reaction to preserve human life. Worry is only classed as a phobia when people
begin to organize their life around either avoiding the important things they are afraid of, or
become highly worried when faced with their phobia.

Research studies on the reasons for phobias have revealed us some info, but almost sufficient
to figure all of it out. Phobias are defined as being irrational fears of certain things or
circumstances so the idea of a fast phobia cure shouldn't take you way too much by surprise.

At this moment we do know that genetics, chemicals in the brain and terrible experiences all
possible play a crucial role. It also appears that there is a connection between a person's fears
and those of their father and mother and other close loved ones. Kids oftentimes learn phobias
from members of the family as they grow up watching the person's response to circumstances
consistently.
We do not have a way to check to see what kinds of phobias we will have now but we do have
several threat aspects that let us know some people have a higher chance of developing one.

Age seems a major part of the determination of when a real phobia will appear. Children
between the ages of 11 to 15 suffer more frequently from social conditions while grownups in
their mid-20 will develop phobias to situational events like crossing bridges or flying in an
aircraft.

Ladies are most likely to show indications of social conditions just because of the simple fact
that guys tend to hide their emotion and stress and anxiety a bit better, normally including
alcohol.

We were born with only 2 fears. The worry of falling and the fear of loud noises. Every other
fear we have learned whilst growing up.

This means that a real phobia is something we have gained from someplace or somebody.
Stressed emotions of any kind are a result of our perceptions. Our perceptions are the result of
our life experiences and the meaning we position upon them. So if you have a serious phobia of

spiders then the worry you feel is a result of your perceptions about spiders. Your perceptions about spiders are a result of all your life experiences with them and the meaning you have attached to those experiences. Any treatments for anxiety in views to phobias must involve the changing of perceptions.

To eliminate anxiety from a particular phobia you must deal with the unconscious mind to release any negative emotion that have been connected to any past experiences with the trigger object. When you ask what phobia means it is just the outcome of the unconscious mind having paired intense levels of worry with the object of the phobia. To call a real phobia a disorder of any kind is to presume that there is something wrong the psychological procedures of the person involved.

Our minds work exactly like a computer system. We can only produce results according to the software we have. Our software is the accumulation of our life experiences and the meanings we have positioned on them.
A real phobia is just a result a person is producing. They had the needed life experiences and applied the required meaning to those experiences to allow them to produce that result. Although we cannot return and change the life experiences we can change the meaning we have applied to those experiences. This creates an automatic change in perception which allows us to change results and acquire stress and anxiety attacks relief.

To alter the meaning we have actually attached to a specific life experience we need to release the negative emotion that has been kept with it. Whenever a particular memory is activated the mind sends out the signal to the appropriate organs of the body so that you can feel the emotions coupled with that memory. When it comes to a distressing memory, whenever this trigger/response process it is effectively recreating and adding evidence to the original trauma. Unless you do something to disrupt this trigger/response system you are predestined to keep repeating the past.

If you have been frightened by spiders in 100 different life experiences then your mind has 100 different pieces of evidence to say that spiders are something to be terrified of. Till you supply irrefutable proof to the mind

That the reverse is actually true it will not let go of the worry and remove anxiety. The only undeniable proof that the mind will accept is to be in a circumstance with a spider where it doesn't feel fear in the body.

For example, you may know that it is safe to be out on a terrace in a high-rise block, but feel frightened to go out on it and even enjoy the view from behind the windows inside the structure. Likewise, you may know that a spider isn't poisonous or that it won't bite you, but this still doesn't decrease your stress and anxiety.

A lot of us have fears about particular things or situations, and this is flawlessly regular. A fear becomes a real phobia if it lasts for more than 6 months, and has a substantial influence on how you live your daily life.

Is a phobia a psychological illness?

Lots of us have worries about particular things or circumstances, and this is perfectly typical. A fear becomes a real phobia if:
the fear runs out proportion to the risk
it lasts for more than six months
it has a considerable effect on how you live your day-to-day life

The Brain throughout Phobias

Some areas of the brain store and recall hazardous or possibly lethal events.
The amygdala in the brain is thought to be connected to the development of phobias.
If an individual faces a similar event in the future in life, those parts of the brain retrieve the demanding memory, sometimes more than once. This causes the body to experience the same reaction.
In a real phobia, the regions of the brain that handle fear and stress keep retrieving the frightening event wrongly.
Researchers have found that phobias are often connected to the amygdala, which lies behind the pituitary gland in the brain. The amygdala can trigger the release of "fight-or-flight" hormonal agents. These put the body and mind in an extremely alert and stressed out state.

How do phobias happen?
Actually, we're on our way back to the old amygdalae again. Unconscious learning is always happening deep in our minds so as to keep us safe. Actually, it's emotional learning. To put it simply, this learning isn't of the intellectual or rational type.

When our ancestors met some intense animal in the forest, their survival instincts would immediately begin at optimal level, in other words, an anxiety attack. This is the kind of learning that produces the instinctive, rapid sort of re-action.

Just expect we needed to rely on our thinking brain. We 'd be back to where we were with the big bear. If we actually had to think knowingly about what to do, the human species would have passed away out a long period of time ago. This sort of learning happens entirely emotionally, therefore bypassing the 'thinking brain.' Way back, if among our ancestors came across a sabre toothed tiger, this immediate phobic reaction was vitally required for their survival.

There are some fairly easy phobias which can be easily treated, such as a worry of pet dogs, bugs, creeping animals, dental practitioners and flying. Some are more intricate though like having a social phobia or agoraphobia, the fear of open or public areas. My friend in the prior example suffered from that and the only place she wanted to be when that occurred was in her home.

Social phobia or social phobia stress and anxiety can be a very limiting worry as it can effect on tons of social situations, just like work, family events such as wedding events, or needing to perform tasks like public speaking. Typically people experiencing a social phobia, are essentially afraid that they will let themselves down or humiliate themselves in public. Some of the milder symptoms are blushing, sweating and breathing heavily.

Phobias do not just influence on a specific type of person. They can happen to anybody irrespective of creed, sex, age or childhood. I know in my own case that when I was more youthful, around the age of eight, I had a bad and agonizing experience with a dental expert. That effected on me to a great extent. It left me with a dental phobia and when I say that, it impacted me to the degree that I would simply not even walk past a dental expert's surgery if I could avoid it. It prevails that simple phobias like this happen in early childhood, and quite often disappear by themselves as the person ages. Sometimes though as in my own case these do trigger problems in the adult years.
Phobias can start at any age and for a variety of reasons but it is fairly certain we aren't born with any phobias, so at some phase in our lives we develop these. For the purpose of treatment of phobias that is a good idea as though they have been developed, they can be treated.

The more complex phobias normally start as we age whereas the social phobias I have discussed typically start during the teenage years and agoraphobia from around 16 to the early twenties. Complex phobias typically can continue for several years, but there are treatments readily available. Sadly, the conventional phobic classification system has shed little light on the real, but covert systems responsible for creating and forming phobic conduct. In simple fact, this Greek and Latin name-calling might have done a good deal of harm.

Why do we have them?

We have them because a real phobia is a survival system, which in fact has 'failed.' Well-meaning people usually try talking phobics out of their fear, but to no avail. Almost always, such an effort will end in failure.

Under normal situations, fear sets off a natural fight-or-flight response that allows animals to respond quickly to risks in their environment. Unreasonable and excessive fear, however, is usually a maladaptive reaction. In humans, an unwarranted, persistent fear of a particular situation or item, referred to as specific phobia, can trigger frustrating distress and disrupt daily life. Particular phobia is among the more common stress and anxiety disorders, impacting an approximated 9 percent of Americans within their lifetime. Common subtypes include worry of small animals, insects, flying, enclosed areas, blood and needles.

For fear to intensify to illogical levels, a combination of hereditary and ecological elements is very likely at play. Estimates of hereditary contributions to specific phobia range from approximately 25 to 65 percent, although we do not know which genes have a leading part. No specific phobia gene has been identified, and it is highly unlikely that a single gene is accountable. Rather variations in several genes might predispose an individual to developing some psychological symptoms and conditions, including particular phobia. When it comes to the environmental part, a person might develop a phobia after a particularly frightening event, particularly if he or she feels out of control.

Even witnessing or finding out about a distressing incident can add to its development. For instance, watching a terrible airplane crash on the news may activate a fear of flying. That said, critical the beginning of the condition can be hard because people tend to do a bad job of recognizing the source of their worries. Our understanding of how and why phobias emerge remains minimal, but we have made great strides in abating them.

Direct exposure treatment, a type of cognitive-behavior therapy, is widely accepted as the most reliable treatment for stress and anxieties and phobias, and the vast bulk of patients complete treatment within 10 sessions. Throughout direct exposure therapy, a person engages with the specific fear to help decrease and eventually overcome it over time. An individual might, for instance, take a look at a picture of the dreadful item or become immersed in the situation he or she hates. Thankfully for those plagued by unreasonable fears, we can deal with a serious phobia rapidly and effectively without always understanding its origin.

How Phobias Are Classified

While there are literally numerous different types of phobias experienced today, there are a few that are more common than others. These include phobias that are social, phobias that are considered to be particular, in addition to phobia that are special or associated to particular areas and the excess or limitations of those spaces. Individuals who struggle with these typical phobia types experience not only a worry that is straight associated to these phobias, but also some awkward symptoms that can trigger physiological and mental stress on the body.
Complex phobias
Complex phobias just like agoraphobia and social phobia can often have a damaging influence on an individual's everyday life and mental wellness.

Agoraphobia typically involves a mix of some interlinked phobias. For instance, somebody with a worry of going outside or leaving their home might also have a worry of being left alone (monophobia) or of spots where they feel trapped (claustrophobia).

The signs experienced by people with agoraphobia can differ in seriousness. For example, some people can feel extremely anxious and anxious if they need to leave their home to go the shops. Others may feel relatively comfortable taking a trip short distances from their home.

If you have a social phobia, the idea of being seen in public or at social events can make you feel scared, restless and susceptible.

Purposefully keeping away from conference people in social situations is a sign of social phobia. In extreme cases of social phobia, just like agoraphobia, some people are too scared to leave their home.
Some treatment options for phobias are readily available, including talking treatments and self-help techniques. Nevertheless, it can typically take some time to conquer a complicated phobia.

1. Social Phobia This kind of phobia is actually a type of anxiety that exists when social experiences and circumstances are come across. These social circumstances can be as simple as those that are encountered on a daily basis. Individuals who experience this find that they are frightened of other ones watching and passing judgments on them. Social phobias are worries of interacting with people or celebrations and agoraphobias are fears of open spaces or public places from where escape is difficult like going shopping malls, public transport structures etc. These individuals are also stressed when it pertains to dealing with embarrassment in public situations. Tons of may be fearful of speaking in front of other ones, or doing other things in front of others, such as eating.

Social anxiety condition is persistent fear of or anxiety about one or more social or performance situations that is out of percentage to the real threat postured by the situation. Common situations that may be anxiety-provoking include meeting people, including complete strangers, talking in conferences or in groups, beginning discussions, talking with authority figures, working, eating or drinking while being observed, going to school, going shopping, being seen in public, using public toilets and public performances like public speaking. Although fret about some of these circumstances are common in the general population, people with social stress and anxiety disorder worry excessively about them at the time and right before and afterwards.

They fear that they will do or say something that they believe will be humiliating or humiliating (such as blushing, sweating, appearing boring or silly, shaking, appearing incompetent, looking restless). Social anxiety condition can have a great influence on an individual's performance, interrupting regular life, hindering social relationships and quality of life and impairing efficiency at work or school. People with the disorder might misuse alcohol or drugs to try to minimize their stress and anxiety (and relieve anxiety).

Children might show their anxiety in different ways from adults: as well as shrinking from interactions, they may be most likely to sob, freeze or have tantrums. They may also be less likely to acknowledge that their worries are unreasonable when they are away from a social circumstances. Particular circumstances that can cause problem for socially restless children and young people include taking part in class activities, requesting help in class, signing up with activities with peers (such as participating in parties or clubs), and being involved in school performances.

Social stress and anxiety disorder has an early median age of beginning (13 years) and is just one of the most persistent stress and anxiety disorders. In spite of the extent of distress and impairment, only about half of those with the disorder ever seek treatment, and those who do generally only seek treatment after 15 twenty years of symptoms. A considerable number of people who develop social stress and anxiety condition in adolescence may recuperate before reaching adulthood. Nevertheless, if the condition has persisted into their adult years, the chance of recovery in the absence of treatment is modest when compared with lots of other typical mental illness.

Reliable psychological and pharmacological interventions for social stress and anxiety condition exist but might not be accessed as a result of poor recognition, insufficient evaluation and restricted awareness or availability of treatments. Social stress and anxiety condition is under-recognized in primary care. When it exists side-by-side with anxiety the depressive episode might be acknowledged without spotting the underlying and more relentless social stress and anxiety condition. The early age of onset means that recognition in academic settings is also challenging.

Some recommendations in this standard have been adjusted from recommendations in other GREAT medical assistance. In these cases the Standard Development Group bewared to preserve the meaning and intent of the initial recommendations. Changes to wording or structure were made to fit the suggestions into this standard. The initial sources of the adjusted suggestions are displayed in the suggestions.
The standard will presume that prescribers will use a drug's summary of item qualities to notify decisions made with individual service users.

This guideline suggests some drugs for indications for which they do not have a UK marketing permission at the date of publication, if there is good proof to support that usage. The prescriber needs to follow relevant professional guidance, taking full duty for the decision. The service user (or those with authority to give authorization on their behalf) should supply educated approval, which should be documented. See Good practice in prescribing and managing medicines and gadgets for more information. Where recommendations have been produced for using drugs outside their licensed indicators (' off-label usage'), these drugs are marked with a footnote in the suggestions.

2. Particular Phobia - I m scared to death of flying, and I never do it any longer. I used to start fearing an aircraft trip a month right before I was because of leave. It was an awful feeling when that aircraft door closed and I felt trapped. My heart would pound, and I would sweat bullets.

When the airplane would start to rise, it just strengthened the gut feeling that I couldn't get out. When I think of flying, I picture myself losing control, flipping out, and climbing the walls, but naturally I never ever did that. I m not afraid of crashing or hitting turbulence. It's just that sensation of being caught. Whenever I've thought of changing jobs, I've needed to believe, Would I be under pressure to fly? These days I only go places where I can drive or take a train. My good friends always point out that I couldn't leave a train taking a trip at high speeds either, so why don't trains bother me? I just tell them it isn't a reasonable worry.

A particular phobia is an intense, illogical worry of something that poses little or no real danger. Some of the more typical particular phobias are focused around closed-in places, heights, escalators, tunnels, highway driving, water, flying, pets, and injuries including blood. Such phobias aren't just severe worry; they are illogical worry of a specific thing. You might have the ability to ski the world's tallest mountains with ease but be not able to exceed the fifth floor of an office complex. While grownups with phobias realize that these fears are illogical, they often find that facing, or perhaps thinking about facing, the feared thing or circumstances brings on a panic attack or extreme anxiety.

Specific phobias affect an approximated 19.2 million adult Americans1 and are twice as typical in ladies as men.10 They normally appear in childhood or teenage years and tend to continue into the adult years.12 The reasons for specific phobias aren't well comprehended, but there is some proof that the tendency to develop them might run in families.

If the feared circumstances or feared thing is easy to stay away from, people with specific phobias may not seek assistance; but if avoidance disrupts their careers or their individual lives, it can become disabling and treatment is generally went after.
Specific phobias respond very well to thoroughly targeted psychotherapy.

A particular phobia includes being afraid of a particular circumstances or thing. When a specific experiences this, they tend to keep away from the item or area that they have a fear of.

The specific phobia is suffered by about a single person out of 10. It can be absolutely anything, but triggered by a specific object or circumstances. The fear is intense. In truth, it's a pan4ic attack. An example of the type of phobia consists of that of Arachnophobia, which is a fear of spiders.

Basic phobias might also be a fear of blood, medical interventions like injections, or injury. Victims might faint in the presence of blood or injury, following a decrease in their heart rate and blood pressure.

This is called a vasovagal reaction which causes fainting. It does not usually occur with other anxiety conditions. In other phobias and panic disorders, the person's heart beat and blood pressure typically increases as their arousal rate boosts.

3. Spatial Fear (A non-specific) - A spatial phobia includes a particular location of the amount of space present. Agoraphobia is a typical phobia which can be defined as a generalized fear of leaving a familiar 'safe' place such as home, and of the possible panic attacks which may follow. It might also be a result of panic attack which in severe cases, avoids sufferers from leaving their homes unless joined by people they rely on. Agoraphobia is derived from a Greek word meaning "worry of the open marketplace".

Agoraphobia is different from panic attack, though lots of people who have panic attack typically suffer from agoraphobia. People who have panic attack go through repeating unforeseeable episodes of serious panic with no particular reason. Due to the intensity of symptoms which mark panic disorders, it is usually mistaken for lethal diseases such as a cardiac arrest. Signs consist of sweating, shortness of breath, hyperventilation, dizziness, unmanageable worry, quick heartbeat, and dizziness.

A non-specific phobia is a fear of a more generalized nature. Agoraphobia, for instance, is non-specific. The worry of open areas, or the more modern-day connected meaning where the worry includes remaining in a congested place.
What many non-sufferers find very tough to understand is that the phobia's fear is so usually of a non-threatening nature. I discussed buttons early on. Who in the world would be afraid of a button, we really wonder? The indicate understand, however, is that phobias have nothing whatever to do with the reasonable thinking part of the brain.
Understand, too, that the poor phobic can extremely typically see the irrationality of their fear themselves. It sounds just as silly to them too, but nevertheless whatever it may be still frightens them.

Chapter 4: Specific Phobias to Mention

Acrophobia - Worry of Heights.

There is an important difference between fear of heights and acrophobia. I think we all have a particular worry of being up high. Worry is a mechanism for preservation. And there is definitely a threat when we find ourselves in a place where a slip in balance could lead us to putting ourselves at threat. So becoming afraid when in such a circumstance is a natural response of protection. It's when just the idea of being in an elevated place elicits an afraid or panicked reaction, then it's likely that you are handling a phobia.

Claustrophobia - Worry of Little Areas

There is a large series of reactions that have been categorized as claustrophobia. So if you start to feel a fear when you crawl into extremely little spaces where you are confined and would have trouble turning around that is one level of fear of small spaces. There is the other end of the spectrum where you feel panic when the door to your room is closed. Again the truly tight space fear can be thought about a regular response to be limited in movement. Again a conservation system, as we are programed with 2 responses to aggressive conduct. One way that we can react is by battling, and the other way is by running. I am sure you can see how being in a confined space would limit your ability to combat, and definitely eliminate your capability to run. So I do not think being in a really confined space is necessarily a phobic reaction, just a natural protective measure.

Nyctophobia - Worry of the Dark
This is a common worry in kids and may extend into adulthood. Just like the two preceding phobias, this is your own protective measure brought to an extreme. Among the primary ways in which we secure ourselves is through our senses. When we use our senses we can identify risk right before it is upon us and take action to ensure that we remain safe and alive. Among our primary senses that we have learned to trust is our sight. Darkness severely restricts our capability to see things. There are animals that have exceptional capabilities to see in the dark, which puts us at a disadvantage when we are faced with that type of challenge.

The issue ends up being more worrisome when, because we can't see plainly, we begin to imagine some truly bad repercussions and we increase our worry response.

So as you can see, these three top phobias are truly regular fears that have been permitted to broaden and control our lives in undesirable and unwanted methods. One of the ways in which you can conquer your worries and phobias is with hypnosis and psychological images. When you take a look at the way these worries and phobias take place, you will see a typical link. They are all based upon our instinctual reaction of fight or flight, and our need to secure ourselves.

They are survival systems that are pre-programmed. The distinction between the phobia and the worry is the extent that you enable your creativity to take hold and magnify that worry to an illogical level with a trigger for instant reaction. When you use hypnosis you can learn to use your imagination more effectively.

A really good hypnotherapist can relieve you of the patterns that you have been practicing and help you to build correct mental imagery that will help you in staying calm and well balanced. It is indeed a widely known simple fact that a ton of individuals have particular kind of phobia, like worry for test or severe anxiety for public speaking.

Simply put, many of us experience a short duration of extreme worry as well as stress and anxiety in certain situations. In even worse cases, there are people who have prolonged phobias that put them under both psychological and physical distress for a prolonged period of time. Keep reading to discover the 3 main classifications of the phobias that are most frequently seen among us.

Brief summary of Phobias:

The fear of:
spiders (Arachnophobia).
social situations (social phobia).
flying (Aviatophobia).
open areas (Agoraphobia).
confined spaces (Claustrophobia).
heights (Acrophobia).
cancer (Cancerophobia).
thunderstorms (worry of lightening astraphobia; worry of thunder Brontophobia).
death (Necrophobia).
heart disease (Cardiophobia).

Another type of phobia which is very common nowadays is the agoraphobia. Bearing a certain degree of similarity to the formerly talked about social phobia, agoraphobia can be defined as the fear of open space. Typically, people who suffer from it would have anxiety attack too, since both signs are actually interconnected. Besides that, they will not be able to go to spots like shopping center, cinemas and so on as they will become panic.

The third category of phobia is simply pointing to the worry of a specific thing, animal, person or perhaps a particular situation. Truth to be told, this classification of phobia is the least severe among all the three classifications that we have discussed. People who suffer from this phobia will only experience anxiety condition when they enter into contact with that particular thing. Normally, this category of phobia is fairly much easier to deal with and many people have successfully overcame their worries through therapy and diagnosis.

Claustrophobia. Agoraphobia. Triskaidekaphobia.

All of these names have one thing in common: they include secret and confusion to what is already one of the most improperly understood aspects of human behavior.

Phobias have always been classified according to their obvious triggers; the items or situations that provoke the worry. These triggers are customarily dressed in exotic Greek and Latin labels, giving each phobia a more clinical air.

Symptoms of a Fear
All phobias can restrict your everyday activities and may cause serious anxiety and anxiety. Complex phobias, such as agoraphobia and social phobia, are most likely to cause these signs.

People with phobias usually intentionally stay away from entering contact with the thing that causes them fear and anxiety. For example, someone with a worry of spiders (arachnophobia) might not want to touch a spider and even look at an image of one.
In many cases, an individual can develop a real phobia where they become afraid of experiencing anxiety itself as it feels so awkward.

You don't have to be in the circumstances you're afraid of to experience the symptoms of phobia The brain is able to develop a response to terrifying circumstances even when you aren't actually in the situation.

The signs of a real phobia include experiencing extreme worry and anxiety when confronted with the situation or object that you are scared of. If your phobia is severe, thinking of the object of your phobia can also activate these signs. If you come near to, or into contact with, the feared circumstances you become anxious or distressed. In addition you may also have one or more undesirable physical symptoms.

An advancement of keeping away from the things of phobias is that this sort of behaviour can result in loss of Self-esteem which can in turn typically reinforce the fear related to the phobia. Frequently this can further turn into anxiety.
Signs of a phobia consist of:

Physical symptoms

People with phobias typically have panic attack. Anxiety attack can be very frightening and traumatic. The signs often happen unexpectedly and without caution.
As well as frustrating feelings of anxiety, a panic attack can trigger physical signs, like:
sweating
shivering

hot flushes or chills
shortness of breath or trouble breathing
a choking sensation
quick heartbeat (tachycardia).
strong pain or tightness in the chest.
an experience of butterflies in the stomach.
nausea.
headeache and lightheadedness.
feeling faint.
tingling or pins and needles.
dry mouth.
a need to go to the toilet.
sounding in your ears.
confusion or disorientation.
feeling unsteady, lightheaded, lightheaded or faint.
feeling like you are choking.
a pounding heart, palpitations or sped up heart rate.
chest pain or tightness in the chest.
hot or cold flushes.
shortness of breath or a smothering experience.
queasiness, vomiting or diarrhea.
tingling or tingling feelings.
trembling or shaking.

The physical signs are partly triggered by the brain which sends out a ton of messages down nerves to numerous parts of the body when you are restless. In addition, you launch tension hormonal agents - such as adrenaline (epinephrine) - into the blood stream when you are anxious. These can also act on the heart, muscles and other parts of the body to cause signs. You might even become anxious by just thinking of the feared situation. You wind up avoiding the feared situation as much as possible, which can limit your life and cause distress.

Mental symptoms.
In extreme cases, you might also experience psychological signs, such as:
fear of losing control.
fear of fainting.
feelings of fear.
fear of dying.
feeling out of touch with reality or detached from your body.

Experiencing this type of severe fear is extremely unpleasant and can be really frightening. It might make you feel stressed, out of control and overwhelmed. It might also lead to feelings of embarrassment, stress and anxiety or anxiety.

As a result, many people with phobias keep away from circumstances where they might have to face their worry. While this is an efficient technique to begin with, avoiding your worries often causes them to worsen, and can start to have a substantial impact on how you live your life.

The Very Best Treatment Methods
Various methods are said to deal with phobias. Their proposed advantages may vary from person to person.
Some therapists use virtual reality or images workout to desensitize clients to the feared entity. These belong to systematic desensitization therapy
Cognitive and behavior modifications help you to change certain ways that you think, feel and behave. They are useful treatments for numerous mental health issue, including phobias.

Cognitive treatment is based upon the idea that certain point of views can activate, or fuel, certain mental illness such as anxiety, anxiety and phobias. The therapist helps you to understand your present idea patterns. In specific, to determine any hazardous, unhelpful and false ideas or mindsets which you have that can make you anxious. The aim is then to change your ways of thinking to stay away from these ideas. Also, to help your thought patterns to be more sensible and helpful.

Behavioral therapy aims to change any behaviors which are harmful or not helpful. For instance, with phobias your response to the feared item (anxiety and avoidance) is not handy. The therapist helps you to change this. Various methods are used, depending upon the condition and situations. For example, for agoraphobia the therapist will normally help you to face up to feared circumstances, a little bit at a time. A first step may be to choose a really brief walk from your home with the therapist who gives support and guidance. In time, a longer walk may be possible, then a walk to the stores, then a trip on a bus, etc. The therapist might teach you how to manage stress and anxiety when you confront the feared circumstances and places. For example, by using deep breathing workouts. This strategy of behavior modification is called direct exposure therapy where you are exposed more and more to feared situations and learn how to cope.

Direct exposure treatment.
Because many phobic conditions include avoidance, direct exposure treatment, a particular psychotherapy, is the treatment of choice. With structure and assistance from a clinician who recommends exposure homework, clients seek out, challenge, and stay in contact with what they fear and stay away from until their anxiety is slowly relieved through a process called habituation. Since most clients know their fears are excessive and might be embarrassed by their fears, they are generally going to participate in this treatment ie, to keep away from staying away from.
Typically, clinicians start with a moderate direct exposure (eg, clients are asked to carefully approach the feared thing). If patients define velocity of their heart rate or shortness of breath

when they encounter the feared circumstances or object, they may be taught to respond with sluggish, controlled breathing or other approaches that promote relaxation. Or, they might be asked to note when their heart rate sped up and shortness of breath began and when these response returned towards typical. When clients feel comfortable at one level of exposure, the direct exposure level is increased (eg, to touching the feared item).

Clinicians continue to increase the direct exposure level until patients can tolerate normal interaction with the circumstances or item (eg, ride in an elevator, cross a bridge). Exposure can increase as rapidly as clients endure it; often just a couple of sessions are needed.

Exposure treatment helps > 90% of patients who carry it out consistently and is almost always the only treatment needed for specific phobias.
Cognitive behavioral therapy (CBT) is a mix of the two where you may take advantage of changing both your thoughts and your conduct s.

CBT is generally done in weekly sessions of about 50 minutes each, for some weeks. You need to take an active part and are given research between sessions. For example, you might be asked to keep a journal of your thoughts which happen when you become restless.

Note: unlike other forms of talking treatments (psychiatric therapy), CBT does not look into the events of the past. CBT aims to handle your existing thought procedures and/or behaviors, and helps to change them where suitable. CBT typically works well to treat most phobias but doesn't suit everyone. Nevertheless, it might not be available on the NHS in all regions.

(CBT) can be helpful. Cognitive behavior modification allows the patient to challenge inefficient ideas or beliefs by bearing in mind their own emotions with the aim that the client will realize their fear is unreasonable. CBT may be conducted in a group setting. Gradual desensitization treatment and CBT are usually effective, offered the client is willing to endure some discomfort. In one medical trial, 90% of patients were observed with no longer having a phobic response after successful CBT treatment.

Antidepressant medications
These are frequently used to deal with anxiety. Nevertheless, they also help to decrease the signs of phobias (particularly agoraphobia and social phobia), even if you are not depressed. They work by interfering with brain chemicals (neurotransmitters) just like serotonin which may be associated with triggering stress and anxiety symptoms.

Antidepressants do not work straightaway. It takes 2 to 4 weeks right before their effect develops and anxiety is helped. A typical problem is that some people stop the medication after a week or so, as they feel that it is doing no good, and it is too early to tell if the medication is working.
Antidepressants are not tranquillizers and are not generally addicting.
There are some kinds of antidepressants, each with numerous benefits and drawbacks and they differ in their possible side-effects. However, selective serotonin reuptake inhibitor (SSRI)

antidepressants are the ones most typically used for stress and anxiety and phobic disorders. Examples of SSRIs are citalopram and sertraline.

Note: after first beginning an antidepressant, in some people stress and anxiety symptoms can become worse for a few days right before they begin to improve. Your physician or practice nurse will want to keep an examine you in the very first weeks of treatment to see how you manage.

A combination of CBT and an SSRI antidepressant may work better in some cases than either treatment alone.

Benzodiazepines

Benzodiazepines such as diazepam are sometimes called small tranquilizers but they can have serious side-effects. They often work well in the short term to relieve symptoms of anxiety. The issue is they are addictive and can lose their effect if you take them for more than several weeks. They might also make you sleepy. Therefore, they are not a useful long-term treatment for phobias. A brief course, or even a single dosage, might be recommended for a phobia which happens hardly ever; however, there is no proof to support this practice. Recommendation for CBT or a fear of flying course (organized by a lot of airlines) is more efficient. Benzodiazepines may work in acute treatment of serious signs but the danger benefit ratio is really against their long term use in phobic disorders.

There are also new pharmacological techniques, which target learning and memory processes that happen throughout psychiatric therapy. For example, it has been shown that glucocorticoids can boost termination based psychotherapy.

Eye Movement Desensitization and Reprocessing

(EMDR) has been demonstrated in peer reviewed medical trials to be effective in treating some phobias. Mainly used to deal with Post traumatic stress condition, EMDR has been shown as effective in alleviating phobia signs following a specific trauma, such as a fear of pets following a dog bite Hypnotherapy combined with Eurolinguistics programs can also be used to help eliminate the associations that activate a phobic reaction.

However, lack of research and scientific testing jeopardizes its status as an efficient treatment.

Psychotherapeutic alternative medicine tool, also thought about to be pseudoscience by the mainstream medicine, is supposedly useful.

Another approach psychologists and psychiatrists use to deal with clients with severe phobias is extended direct exposure. Prolonged direct exposure is used in psychotherapy when the person with the phobia is exposed to the item of their fear over a long period of time. when an individual has overcome avoidance of or leave from the phobic item or situation. People with minor distress from their phobias usually do not need extended direct exposure to their worry.

These treatment choices aren't equally exclusive. Usually a therapist will suggest multiple treatments.

Efficient and Safe Herbal Remedies for Phobias

Whatever might be the reason there are effective natural treatments for phobia just like ginseng, lemon or lime, valerian root or lavender oil.

Lemon or Lime: The juice of a lemon or lime works for lowering lightheadedness or queasiness associated with a real phobia. Just cut a lemon into 2 halves and smell it for getting relief during an attack of phobia.

Ginseng: This herb is known for its stimulating and unwinding homes and is used thoroughly for the treatment of nerves.

Valerian Root: This herb can be used for the treatment of sleeping disorders. It has the homes for relaxing the nerves and the central nervous system of an agitated person and therefore is used as an efficient herbal remedy for the treatment of phobia. Grind 5-6 valerian roots for preparing the herbal remedy. It should be taken in 2-3 times a day for decreasing the impacts of phobia. However, pregnant and nursing mothers should stay away from the usage of the powder of valerian root.

Lavender: This is another reliable solution for phobia. Lavender has a soothing influence on the body and has an enjoyable odor. Daily lavender oil massage can help in eliminating an attack of phobia. The best way to lower stress is by including drops of lavender oil to the bathing water for a relaxing bath.

Kava: This is a well-known herb used for treating and sedating psychological clients. It relaxes the mind without hampering the mental clearness of the patients. Taking in the kava herb day-to-day builds up the tolerance level that is valuable in reducing phobia. The basic everyday dose of kava is 250 mg.

Passion Flower: The passion flower is a reliable natural extract that increases the performance of the nervous system and brain and helps to keep the organs in a healthy equilibrium. This natural treatment works in controlling phobias and panic.

Supragya Plus: In addition to the organic and natural remedies, there are certain ayurvedic solutions for phobia. Supragya plus is one such nerve tonic that strengthens the nerves and solves the nerve associated problems that consist of depression, stress and anxiety, phobia, stress, irritability, anger, intolerance, sleeplessness, palpitation and a lot more.

Ashwagandha: This is another efficient ayurvedic remedy that can be used in the treatment depression, stress and anxiety and other psychiatric conditions related with a phobia. The leaves, roots, and berries of the herb have medical residential or commercial properties that prove to be effective in the treatment of an array of mental disorders.

Phobia is a serious mental disorder but with a healthy diet, correct workout and certain natural and ayurvedic treatments the issue can be successfully handled.

Getting rid of Phobias

While people might be amused by a good friend or family member shouting at the sight of a mouse or incapacitated with worry throughout a thunderstorm, phobias are no laughing matter for those whose lives are being adversely impacted. Fortunately, is that phobias are common and treatable and that comprehending a serious phobia is the primary step to overcoming it.

A Normal Fear vs. a Phobia

Fear is necessary to our survival. When we're scared, our primitive, automated fight or flight response is triggered. Afferent neuron fire in the brain and chemicals like adrenaline, noradrenaline and cortisol are released into our blood stream. In reaction, our breathing rate increases so we have trouble breathing. Blood is diverted from our digestive system to our limb muscles so our hearts pound and our stomachs churn. Our awareness intensifies. Our sight sharpens. Our impulses accelerate. We're now prepared to stand our ground and battle or run for our lives. Our forefathers needed this response to fight intruders or leave wild animals and it's just as essential today.

This reaction helps us make flash decisions to avert things like car accidents and sharpens our mental acuity so we can do things like meet abrupt due dates.

A fear has been referred to as a worry on steroids. For instance, it's regular to fear a snarling tiger. It's a real phobia, when you experience the same reaction fear when confronted by a friendly house cat.

There are many strategies to help get rid of phobias. Some you can try yourself and others need expert assistance. If your phobia is so severe that it sets off regular panic attacks and is negatively impacting your quality of your life, think about professional counselling.
Whether you're receiving professional aid or not, self-help strategies can make you feel more in control and that is the initial step to dominating any worry.

Here are several:

Relaxation methods.
Relaxation strategies such as deep breathing, meditation, and muscle relaxation are great ways to help you cope better with any stress and stress and anxiety in your life. With routine practice, they can enhance your ability to control the physical signs of anxiety, which will make facing your phobia less intimidating.

Challenging negative thoughts.
Altering distorted thinking patterns is part of what therapists call Cognitive Behavioral Therapy (CBT). The theory behind CBT is that our thinking (cognitive) affects the way we act (behavioral) and that by changing our thinking we can change our conduct. With phobias this requires determining and taking a look at negative beliefs that develop the distorted thought patterns that make us feel afraid.

These ideas are then challenged and changed with more realistic ones. For example, All pet dogs are vicious and will injure me. That idea is analyzed (what is the proof?) and challenged (that declaration is a gross overgeneralization) and ultimately changed with Not all canines are vicious. Most are kind and won't harm me.

Slowly facing your worries.
It makes sense to keep away from an object or situation that causes an intense and unpleasant response. However, that doesn't aid to conquer a serious phobia. Gradually facing your fear teaches your brain that your phobia might not be so frightening after all.
Many easy phobias can be effectively dealt with using a form of behavior modification referred to as exposure therapy or desensitization and can be finished with a therapist or without. It's done gradually. Each small step is repeated until the fear and stress and anxiety decreases. Only when you feel in control do you transfer to the next step.

For example, if you are scared of elevators, you may try the following steps:
1. Spend one minute in front of elevator doors.
2. Spend one minute checking out an elevator.
3. Spend one minute in an unmoving elevator with the door open.

For serious and complex concerns, desensitization treatment can take a considerable amount of time, but works well for less serious phobias.

There are also different medications available to help people deal with anxiety and these are usually used in conjunction with other treatments by medical occupations. So if your phobia continues to have an unfavorable influence on your life, connect for assistance. Phobias can be overcome often rapidly so there's no need to live your life in fear.

Interesting facts about phobias.
Phobias are more serious than simple fear experiences and are not restricted to fears of particular triggers.
Regardless of individuals knowing that their phobia is illogical, they cannot control the fear reaction.
Signs might include sweating, chest discomforts, and pins and needles.
Treatment can include medication and behavior modification.
Usually, particular phobias start in childhood, between 7 to eleven years with many cases starting before age 10.
Roughly 5% of kids and 16% of teenagers will have a specific phobia in their life time.
Girls are more likely to experience a serious phobia than boys at a rate of 2:1.
Fears are different than typical childhood worries. While kids normally become less scared of things like strangers, the bath, or the boogie beast, as they grow, kids with phobias usually become more scared as they mature. In addition, phobias hardly ever disappear by themselves. Phobias do not reduce with suitable reassurance and provision of info. For example, a dog phobia continues in spite of telling your child that grandmas dog is kind, has no teeth to bite because it is old, and will not scratch.

Some Reasons for a Phobia

Genetic and ecological factors can cause phobias. Children who have a close relative with a stress and anxiety condition are at threat of developing a phobia. Traumatic events, like almost drowning, can induce a serious phobia. Direct exposure to restricted spaces, severe heights, and animal or insect bites can all be sources of phobias.

People with ongoing medical conditions or health concerns usually have phobias. There's a high occurrence of people developing phobias after distressing brain injuries. Drug abuse and depression are also connected to phobias. Fears have different symptoms from serious mental illnesses such as schizophrenia. In schizophrenia, people have visual and acoustic hallucinations, deceptions, fear, negative signs like an hedonic, and disorganized signs. Fears may be irrational, but people with phobias do not fail reality screening.

A phobia is a fear, a worry that for many people is incapacitating and life changing. But let's just explore the entire concept of fear for a 2nd. Fear is great. Worry is a feeling that protects us when we are in risk. Think of a world without any worry, and you imagine a world of lawlessness and anarchy. Without fear, we would have little or no reward to behave and safeguard ourselves. Worry is our brain's way of safeguarding us.

Throughout the ages we have learned to be scared of certain things and situations. It is worry that secures us from snakes, sharks, and situations that can hurt us. We are right to be afraid of serpents-- lots of them are venomous and even if they don't kill us, we know that at finest we will feel pain. Similarly, we know that if we fall from a great height, the chances are we will break a leg or potentially die. So, in these circumstances we are right to feel fear, as it secures us.

Many people don't particularly like spiders or serpents, but they don't struggle with a major phobia. So when does a normal worry become a real phobia, and what causes some people to develop a real phobia of daily circumstances and things?

The answer to what causes a serious phobia is specific to each person, but certain circumstances may contribute to the circumstances. For instance, an individual who experiences a panic attack in an elevator might avoid taking an elevator after that for fear of experiencing another panic attack, in spite of the simple fact that the environment probably played no role in the initial
attack. The individual will, maybe unconsciously, blame the elevator for the attack, and ultimately the elevator and the anxiety attack ended up being so interlinked, that quickly a worry of elevators and confined areas has developed, and the individual now suffers from claustrophobia.

A serious phobia may also be inherited, or rather taught. Take the case of Brian, an 11yr old boy who is afraid of flying. Why is an 11yr old so scared of flying? The answer might be that his mother is also scared. We learn much from our mother and father, and trust them to protect us. Therefore, if our parent, who is supposed to protect us, is scared of something, we learn that it must be damaging and that we too should hesitate of it. The huge risk here is that what may be a moderate fear in a moms and dad, can turn into a full incapacitating phobia in a child.

The just one thing that all phobias have in common is that they are psychological, and for that reason the treatment of phobias lies there. By understanding why we experience a particular phobia, we can begin to treat it. One of the best ways of dealing with phobias is with hypnosis. Hypnosis works by re-training the mind subconsciously to react to the phobia in a different way. By doing it subconsciously, a great deal of the stress and stress and anxiety is taken out of the treatment for the client-- for lots of people, even speaking about their phobia can cause extreme stress.

Just one thing that everybody who conquers their phobia has in common is a big sense of relief. When we face up to, and overcome our worries we begin to realize how we have been held back, and the enormous sense of liberty is overwhelming. That doesn't mean that phobias can be considered minor or banal-- they're far from it. For sufferers, they are very real, and all consuming. At http://www.free-hypnosisdownloads.com there is a growing number of outstanding hypnosis mp3 downloads that help victims of various kinds of phobias to conquer them easily and quickly. The download sessions usually last about 30-40mins to listen to, and their success rate is rather incredible.

Hypnosis is so effective in the treatment of phobias since it addresses the phobia in precisely the same way that it got there in the first place-- subconsciously. This makes the entire experience so much more satisfying for the topic, and for that reason the likelihood of success is incredibly high.

Social Phobias

When an individual is extremely awkward and also has severe amounts of anxiety concerning social situations, it is called social stress and anxiety. It is also described as social phobia and is a disorder. These people constantly have the fear of being judged, watched or slammed. These people have such a great amount of worry that it does disrupt life at school, work, and any kind of social activity or perhaps with everyday life. The majority of these people do understand that the fear is something that is not actually needed but are still not able to stop it.

Social phobia is also one form of phobia. A few people feel afraid to drink or even eat in front of other individuals. Some of them do not speak in front of other people also. Some of the cases may be so extreme that the person is terrified to speak to another person. Physical symptoms develop in a lot of the cases of social phobia. They include blushing, sweating, talking with problem, palpitations, trembling, discomfort in the stomach and many more. It makes it very basic if they deal with these issues rather than fretting more about it.

Social phobia might be triggered because of many a reason. In might be just because of the simple fact that it runs in the family. Therefore, the children get the exact same problems from their mom and dad. It may also be due to alcoholism or due to depression. In women social depression happens two times as much as men for reasons which we do not know. It may start at youth or perhaps at adolescence. It hardly ever begins at 25 years of age. Researches have been going on in this field to learn all the problems that are causing social phobia.

Some of the researchers have been blaming the cause if these signs on a small structure present in the brain which is called amygdale. Our sense of worry is what is controlled by this amygdale. Another group of scientists really believe that this social phobia is passed down from generation to generation.

Yet another group of researchers say that the reason for this social phobia is because of a sensitivity that is very high to disapproval, it may also be based upon physiological reasons or on hormones.

The environment may be yet another reason for the reason for social phobia according to a few researchers. This may be because of something that happened to another person in the same situation. It is called observational learning. This simply put is learning to behave based upon others around you.

Environmental and genetic elements result in phobias. Kids who are prone to anxiety conditions are at a higher danger of developing these phobias. Extreme heights, restricted areas, exposure to insect or animal bites or an upsetting event like near drowning could be a source of such phobias. Even those people with chronic medical conditions just like drug abuse, anxiety or brain injuries are prone to developing these phobias.

Throughout the last few decades, scientists, psychologists and doctors have investigated and analyzed lots of people who struggle with different kinds of Phobia. The very first thing to keep in mind here is once more that Phobias are incredibly complex and there is no chance to tell with 100% certainty that someone is experiencing a phobia.
Phobias-banner-zafirides2

However, there are clear signs that most of phobias develop throughout early childhood, teenage years or early adulthood. It is rather unusual for a serious phobia to develop out of absolutely nowhere after the age of 30 35. Phobias can be brought on by difficult circumstances, certain experiences or frightening events. It is also understood that kids can develop the same phobia among their parents struggled with if they were progressively aware of this during childhood.

Causes for the Simple Phobias

Specific (or simple) phobias often appear to develop in early childhood between the ages of 4 and 8 years of age. Certain events in life or unpleasant experiences can usually plant a seed, which will grow overtime and slowly develop into some sort of phobia. For instance, an undesirable experience in a confined (or small) space could possibly cause claustrophobia in a later stage of life.

Doctors have found that phobias aren't always genetically acquired from either of the mom and dad. However, if a child is progressively aware of one of its father and mother phobia, chances are much higher that this child will develop the exact same (or a similar) phobia during later phases in life. For instance, if a mother experiences Arachnophobia (worry of spiders) then it is far more very likely for her daughter to develop the exact same phobia as well, simply since she was highly aware of her mom's fear throughout childhood.

Causes for Complex Phobias

Like the name suggests, the causes for complex and/or social phobias are still shrouded in clouds of mystery and uncertainty. Scientists believe that the complex phobias are typically triggered by a combination of genetics, brain chemistry and certain life experiences. It is said that social phobias are more likely to be brought on by a very demanding experience than agoraphobia.

Some say that there may be an evolutionary clarification for some kinds of phobias. In age-old times for example, staying outdoors in a wide and open field would increase the risk of getting caught by other unsafe predators. For that reason, it's only logical that for lots of people, specifically for young children, there is a strong instinct for staying safe in the house.

Furthermore, today's social phobias could have been a potential survival instinct in old times. Staying with a group of complete strangers (people from another tribe perhaps) was far more hazardous countless years ago than it is now. Very few people today in a congested mall will want to battle you over your newly caught deer.

Another highly acceptable cause for complicated phobias might be found in the field of neuroscience. Some areas of the brain (see image) are understood to store info about dangerous and even fatal events. If a similar event is faced at some point in the future, the brain will automatically recall those old memories and make the body react as if it were a recurrence. As phobias are irrational phenomena, in some cases it's possible to deal with victims by managing to get the brain to change the bad and negative memories of certain events with something more rational and rational. Nevertheless, the parts of the brain that handle worry typically keep recovering the bad memories. This makes it very difficult to find an extremely effective medical treatment for complicated phobias.

Much is still unidentified about the real reason for some phobias. Causes may also include:

Tons of phobias develop as a result of having a negative experience or panic attack related to a specific thing or situation.

There may be a link between your own specific phobia and the phobia or stress and anxiety of your father and mother this could be as a result of genetics or learned behavior.

Changes in brain working also may play a role in developing particular phobias.

Danger elements
These aspects might increase your threat of particular phobias:

Your age.
Particular phobias can first appear in childhood, usually by age 10, but can occur later in life.

Your relatives.
If somebody in your family has a specific phobia or anxiety, you're more likely to develop it, too. This could be an acquired propensity, or kids might learn particular phobias by observing a family member's phobic response to a things or a scenario.

Your temperament.
Your threat may increase if you're more sensitive, more hindered or more negative than the norm.

An unfavorable experience.
Experiencing a frightening terrible event, such as being trapped in an elevator or attacked by an animal, might set off the development of a specific phobia.

Finding out about negative experiences.
Hearing about negative information or experiences, such as airplane crashes, can result in the development of a particular phobia.

Problems

Although specific phobias may appear ridiculous to other ones, they can be devastating to the people who have them, triggering issues that impact many aspects of life.

Social isolation. Staying away from spots and things you fear can trigger academic, professional and relationship problems. Children with these disorders are at threat of scholastic issues and solitude, and they might have trouble with social skills if their habits considerably differ from their peers.
Mood conditions. Many people with particular phobias have depression in addition to other stress and anxiety disorders.
Substance abuse. The tension of living with an extreme particular phobia may cause abuse of drugs or alcohol.
Suicide. Some people with specific phobias may be at danger of suicide.

Environmental and hereditary elements lead to phobias. Kids who are vulnerable to anxiety disorders are at a greater danger of developing these phobias. Extreme heights, confined spaces, direct exposure to insect or animal bites or a distressing event like near drowning could be a source of such phobias. Even those people with persistent medical conditions like substance abuse, depression or brain injuries are susceptible to developing these phobias.

It is uncommon for a phobia to begin after the age of 30 years, and the majority of start throughout early youth, the teenage years, or early their adult years.

They can be caused by a demanding experience, a frightening event, or a moms and dad or household member with a real phobia that a kid can 'learn.'

There doesn't seem to be one particular reason for phobias, but there are some factors that might play a crucial role:

Specific incidents or injuries. For example, somebody who experiences a ton of turbulence on an aircraft at a young age may later develop a serious phobia about flying.
Learned responses, picked up in early life. Factors in the family environment, such as parents who are very anxious or restless, can have an impact on the way you manage anxiety in later life. You might develop the exact same particular phobia as a parent or older sibling.

Genetics. Some research suggests that some people are more susceptible to developing a phobia than others.

Reactions to stress or fear. If you have a strong response (or panic attack) in response to a specific situation or object, and you find this humiliating or people around you react strongly, it can trigger you to develop more intense stress and anxiety about being in that situation again. Long-term stress can cause emotions of anxiety and depression and minimize your ability to cope in specific circumstances. This can make you feel more afraid or restless about being in those situations again and, over a long period, could lead to you developing a serious phobia.

Social and particular phobias in some cases run in families, providing proof of a genetic connection. Some people are born with a predisposition towards stress and anxiety, which makes them especially susceptible to developing phobias.

Phobias might develop as a reaction to pressure or following terrible events. In other cases, unreasonable fears might develop with no evident trigger. Adults usually recognize that their worries are unreasonable or excessive, and this can serve as a separating factor. The impacted person may not speak with friends and family about a fear that they actually believe is ridiculous.

Phobias are also a natural part of development. A lot of kids go through phases where they are scared of the dark, of monsters, or of strangers. A lot of teens develop stress and anxieties associated with self-image and other ones' understanding of them.

While these fears are normal and often get left behind gradually, they can sometimes persist or become incapacitating.

Everybody has things that terrify them. Nevertheless, there are some people who have strong, irrational, and involuntary responses to everyday things and places, which are called phobias.

There have been some studies examining the causes of phobias, but there is still no real consensus regarding why some people have this type of reaction to certain stimuli. Fears are probably more typical than you may believe according to the National Institutes of Mental Health and the American Psychiatric Association, about 7 to 9 percent of adults in the United States struggle with a particular phobia.

Twenty-one percent of those adults suffer from serious phobias, which translates to about 2 percent of the entire population. Many phobias can be linked to a particular event or situation in the formative years of childhood, but it's not always clear what triggers these phobias.

In most cases, specific phobias develop in early youth between the ages of 7 and 11, though it is possible for a phobia to develop at any age. Particular phobias can be brought on by a variety of different aspects: experiencing a distressing event (e.g. being attacked by a pet dog); observing other ones going through a distressing event (e.g. witnessing a car accident); an unforeseen anxiety attack (e.g. while flying in an airplane); or informative transmittal (e.g. substantial media coverage of a terrorist attack).

Usually, those affected by a specific phobia are not able to identify the reason why their phobia developed. While the cause of a particular phobia may be unidentified, it is necessary to recognize the symptoms and remember that phobias can be treatable if you look for aid from a mental health specialist.

Phobias

What Are Phobias?

A real phobia is a severe form of fear or stress and anxiety activated by a particular
Circumstances (such as going outside) or item (such as spiders), even when There is no risk.

Phobia is basically just an irrational fear of something. In today's society it is easy to find at least
one phobia for every single person you encounter. What triggers phobias though is still an often
pondered question.

Phobias should not be puzzled with easy worries, like being afraid of a lion as that is a normal
protective reaction to preserve human life. Worry is only classed as a phobia when people
begin to organize their life around either avoiding the important things they are afraid of, or
become highly worried when faced with their phobia.

Research studies on the reasons for phobias have revealed us some info, but almost sufficient
to figure all of it out. Phobias are defined as being irrational fears of certain things or
circumstances so the idea of a fast phobia cure shouldn't take you way too much by surprise.

At this moment we do know that genetics, chemicals in the brain and terrible experiences all
possible play a crucial role. It also appears that there is a connection between a person's fears
and those of their father and mother and other close loved ones. Kids oftentimes learn phobias
from members of the family as they grow up watching the person's response to circumstances
consistently.
We do not have a way to check to see what kinds of phobias we will have now but we do have
several threat aspects that let us know some people have a higher chance of developing one.

Age seems a major part of the determination of when a real phobia will appear. Children
between the ages of 11 to 15 suffer more frequently from social conditions while grownups in
their mid-20 will develop phobias to situational events like crossing bridges or flying in an
aircraft.

Ladies are most likely to show indications of social conditions just because of the simple fact
that guys tend to hide their emotion and stress and anxiety a bit better, normally including
alcohol.

We were born with only 2 fears. The worry of falling and the fear of loud noises. Every other
fear we have learned whilst growing up.

This means that a real phobia is something we have gained from someplace or somebody.
Stressed emotions of any kind are a result of our perceptions. Our perceptions are the result of
our life experiences and the meaning we position upon them. So if you have a serious phobia of
spiders then the worry you feel is a result of your perceptions about spiders. Your perceptions

about spiders are a result of all your life experiences with them and the meaning you have attached to those experiences. Any treatments for anxiety in views to phobias must involve the changing of perceptions.

To eliminate anxiety from a particular phobia you must deal with the unconscious mind to release any negative emotion that have been connected to any past experiences with the trigger object. When you ask what phobia means it is just the outcome of the unconscious mind having paired intense levels of worry with the object of the phobia. To call a real phobia a disorder of any kind is to presume that there is something wrong the psychological procedures of the person involved.

Our minds work exactly like a computer system. We can only produce results according to the software we have. Our software is the accumulation of our life experiences and the meanings we have positioned on them.
A real phobia is just a result a person is producing. They had the needed life experiences and applied the required meaning to those experiences to allow them to produce that result. Although we cannot return and change the life experiences we can change the meaning we have applied to those experiences. This creates an automatic change in perception which allows us to change results and acquire stress and anxiety attacks relief.

To alter the meaning we have actually attached to a specific life experience we need to release the negative emotion that has been kept with it. Whenever a particular memory is activated the mind sends out the signal to the appropriate organs of the body so that you can feel the emotions coupled with that memory. When it comes to a distressing memory, whenever this trigger/response process it is effectively recreating and adding evidence to the original trauma. Unless you do something to disrupt this trigger/response system you are predestined to keep repeating the past.

If you have been frightened by spiders in 100 different life experiences then your mind has 100 different pieces of evidence to say that spiders are something to be terrified of. Till you supply irrefutable proof to the mind

That the reverse is actually true it will not let go of the worry and remove anxiety. The only undeniable proof that the mind will accept is to be in a circumstance with a spider where it doesn't feel fear in the body.

For example, you may know that it is safe to be out on a terrace in a high-rise block, but feel frightened to go out on it and even enjoy the view from behind the windows inside the structure. Likewise, you may know that a spider isn't poisonous or that it won't bite you, but this still doesn't decrease your stress and anxiety.

A lot of us have fears about particular things or situations, and this is flawlessly regular. A fear becomes a real phobia if it lasts for more than 6 months, and has a substantial influence on how you live your daily life.

Is a phobia a psychological illness?

Lots of us have worries about particular things or circumstances, and this is perfectly typical. A fear becomes a real phobia if:
the fear runs out proportion to the risk
it lasts for more than six months
it has a considerable effect on how you live your day-to-day life

The Brain throughout Phobias

Some areas of the brain store and recall hazardous or possibly lethal events.
The amygdala in the brain is thought to be connected to the development of phobias.
If an individual faces a similar event in the future in life, those parts of the brain retrieve the demanding memory, sometimes more than once. This causes the body to experience the same reaction.
In a real phobia, the regions of the brain that handle fear and stress keep retrieving the frightening event wrongly.
Researchers have found that phobias are often connected to the amygdala, which lies behind the pituitary gland in the brain. The amygdala can trigger the release of "fight-or-flight" hormonal agents. These put the body and mind in an extremely alert and stressed out state.

How do phobias happen?
Actually, we're on our way back to the old amygdalae again. Unconscious learning is always happening deep in our minds so as to keep us safe. Actually, it's emotional learning. To put it simply, this learning isn't of the intellectual or rational type.

When our ancestors met some intense animal in the forest, their survival instincts would immediately begin at optimal level, in other words, an anxiety attack. This is the kind of learning that produces the instinctive, rapid sort of re-action.

Just expect we needed to rely on our thinking brain. We 'd be back to where we were with the big bear. If we actually had to think knowingly about what to do, the human species would have passed away out a long period of time ago. This sort of learning happens entirely emotionally, therefore bypassing the 'thinking brain.' Way back, if among our ancestors came across a sabre toothed tiger, this immediate phobic reaction was vitally required for their survival.

There are some fairly easy phobias which can be easily treated, such as a worry of pet dogs, bugs, creeping animals, dental practitioners and flying. Some are more intricate though like having a social phobia or agoraphobia, the fear of open or public areas. My friend in the prior example suffered from that and the only place she wanted to be when that occurred was in her home.

Social phobia or social phobia stress and anxiety can be a very limiting worry as it can effect on tons of social situations, just like work, family events such as wedding events, or needing to perform tasks like public speaking. Typically people experiencing a social phobia, are essentially afraid that they will let themselves down or humiliate themselves in public. Some of the milder symptoms are blushing, sweating and breathing heavily.

Phobias do not just influence on a specific type of person. They can happen to anybody irrespective of creed, sex, age or childhood. I know in my own case that when I was more youthful, around the age of eight, I had a bad and agonizing experience with a dental expert. That effected on me to a great extent. It left me with a dental phobia and when I say that, it impacted me to the degree that I would simply not even walk past a dental expert's surgery if I could avoid it. It prevails that simple phobias like this happen in early childhood, and quite often disappear by themselves as the person ages. Sometimes though as in my own case these do trigger problems in the adult years.
Phobias can start at any age and for a variety of reasons but it is fairly certain we aren't born with any phobias, so at some phase in our lives we develop these. For the purpose of treatment of phobias that is a good idea as though they have been developed, they can be treated.

The more complex phobias normally start as we age whereas the social phobias I have discussed typically start during the teenage years and agoraphobia from around 16 to the early twenties. Complex phobias typically can continue for several years, but there are treatments readily available. Sadly, the conventional phobic classification system has shed little light on the real, but covert systems responsible for creating and forming phobic conduct. In simple fact, this Greek and Latin name-calling might have done a good deal of harm.

Why do we have them?

We have them because a real phobia is a survival system, which in fact has 'failed.' Well-meaning people usually try talking phobics out of their fear, but to no avail. Almost always, such an effort will end in failure.

Under normal situations, fear sets off a natural fight-or-flight response that allows animals to respond quickly to risks in their environment. Unreasonable and excessive fear, however, is usually a maladaptive reaction. In humans, an unwarranted, persistent fear of a particular situation or item, referred to as specific phobia, can trigger frustrating distress and disrupt daily life. Particular phobia is among the more common stress and anxiety disorders, impacting an approximated 9 percent of Americans within their lifetime. Common subtypes include worry of small animals, insects, flying, enclosed areas, blood and needles.

For fear to intensify to illogical levels, a combination of hereditary and ecological elements is very likely at play. Estimates of hereditary contributions to specific phobia range from approximately 25 to 65 percent, although we do not know which genes have a leading part. No specific phobia gene has been identified, and it is highly unlikely that a single gene is accountable. Rather variations in several genes might predispose an individual to developing some psychological symptoms and conditions, including particular phobia. When it comes to the environmental part, a person might develop a phobia after a particularly frightening event, particularly if he or she feels out of control.

Even witnessing or finding out about a distressing incident can add to its development. For instance, watching a terrible airplane crash on the news may activate a fear of flying. That said, critical the beginning of the condition can be hard because people tend to do a bad job of recognizing the source of their worries. Our understanding of how and why phobias emerge remains minimal, but we have made great strides in abating them.

Direct exposure treatment, a type of cognitive-behavior therapy, is widely accepted as the most reliable treatment for stress and anxieties and phobias, and the vast bulk of patients complete treatment within 10 sessions. Throughout direct exposure therapy, a person engages with the specific fear to help decrease and eventually overcome it over time. An individual might, for instance, take a look at a picture of the dreadful item or become immersed in the situation he or she hates. Thankfully for those plagued by unreasonable fears, we can deal with a serious phobia rapidly and effectively without always understanding its origin.

How Phobias Are Classified

While there are literally numerous different types of phobias experienced today, there are a few that are more common than others. These include phobias that are social, phobias that are considered to be particular, in addition to phobia that are special or associated to particular areas and the excess or limitations of those spaces. Individuals who struggle with these typical phobia types experience not only a worry that is straight associated to these phobias, but also some awkward symptoms that can trigger physiological and mental stress on the body.
Complex phobias
Complex phobias just like agoraphobia and social phobia can often have a damaging influence on an individual's everyday life and mental wellness.

Agoraphobia typically involves a mix of some interlinked phobias. For instance, somebody with a worry of going outside or leaving their home might also have a worry of being left alone (monophobia) or of spots where they feel trapped (claustrophobia).

The signs experienced by people with agoraphobia can differ in seriousness. For example, some people can feel extremely anxious and anxious if they need to leave their home to go the shops. Others may feel relatively comfortable taking a trip short distances from their home.

If you have a social phobia, the idea of being seen in public or at social events can make you feel scared, restless and susceptible.

Purposefully keeping away from conference people in social situations is a sign of social phobia. In extreme cases of social phobia, just like agoraphobia, some people are too scared to leave their home.

Some treatment options for phobias are readily available, including talking treatments and self-help techniques. Nevertheless, it can typically take some time to conquer a complicated phobia.

1. Social Phobia This kind of phobia is actually a type of anxiety that exists when social experiences and circumstances are come across. These social circumstances can be as simple as those that are encountered on a daily basis. Individuals who experience this find that they are frightened of other ones watching and passing judgments on them. Social phobias are worries of interacting with people or celebrations and agoraphobias are fears of open spaces or public places from where escape is difficult like going shopping malls, public transport structures etc. These individuals are also stressed when it pertains to dealing with embarrassment in public situations. Tons of may be fearful of speaking in front of other ones, or doing other things in front of others, such as eating.

Social anxiety condition is persistent fear of or anxiety about one or more social or performance situations that is out of percentage to the real threat postured by the situation. Common situations that may be anxiety-provoking include meeting people, including complete strangers, talking in conferences or in groups, beginning discussions, talking with authority figures, working, eating or drinking while being observed, going to school, going shopping, being seen in public, using public toilets and public performances like public speaking. Although fret about some of these circumstances are common in the general population, people with social stress and anxiety disorder worry excessively about them at the time and right before and afterwards.

They fear that they will do or say something that they believe will be humiliating or humiliating (such as blushing, sweating, appearing boring or silly, shaking, appearing incompetent, looking restless). Social anxiety condition can have a great influence on an individual's performance, interrupting regular life, hindering social relationships and quality of life and impairing efficiency at work or school. People with the disorder might misuse alcohol or drugs to try to minimize their stress and anxiety (and relieve anxiety).

Children might show their anxiety in different ways from adults: as well as shrinking from interactions, they may be most likely to sob, freeze or have tantrums. They may also be less likely to acknowledge that their worries are unreasonable when they are away from a social circumstance. Particular circumstances that can cause problem for socially restless children and young people include taking part in class activities, requesting help in class, signing up with activities with peers (such as participating in parties or clubs), and being involved in school performances.

Social stress and anxiety disorder has an early median age of beginning (13 years) and is just one of the most persistent stress and anxiety disorders. In spite of the extent of distress and impairment, only about half of those with the disorder ever seek treatment, and those who do generally only seek treatment after 15 twenty years of symptoms. A considerable number of people who develop social stress and anxiety condition in adolescence may recuperate before reaching adulthood. Nevertheless, if the condition has persisted into their adult years, the chance of recovery in the absence of treatment is modest when compared with lots of other typical mental illness.

Reliable psychological and pharmacological interventions for social stress and anxiety condition exist but might not be accessed as a result of poor recognition, insufficient evaluation and restricted awareness or availability of treatments. Social stress and anxiety condition is under-recognized in primary care. When it exists side-by-side with anxiety the depressive episode might be acknowledged without spotting the underlying and more relentless social stress and anxiety condition. The early age of onset means that recognition in academic settings is also challenging.

Some recommendations in this standard have been adjusted from recommendations in other GREAT medical assistance. In these cases the Standard Development Group bewared to preserve the meaning and intent of the initial recommendations. Changes to wording or structure were made to fit the suggestions into this standard. The initial sources of the adjusted suggestions are displayed in the suggestions.
The standard will presume that prescribers will use a drug's summary of item qualities to notify decisions made with individual service users.

This guideline suggests some drugs for indications for which they do not have a UK marketing permission at the date of publication, if there is good proof to support that usage. The prescriber needs to follow relevant professional guidance, taking full duty for the decision. The service user (or those with authority to give authorization on their behalf) should supply educated approval, which should be documented. See Good practice in prescribing and managing medicines and gadgets for more information. Where recommendations have been produced for using drugs outside their licensed indicators (' off-label usage'), these drugs are marked with a footnote in the suggestions.

2. Particular Phobia - I m scared to death of flying, and I never do it any longer. I used to start fearing an aircraft trip a month right before I was because of leave. It was an awful feeling when that aircraft door closed and I felt trapped. My heart would pound, and I would sweat bullets.

When the airplane would start to rise, it just strengthened the gut feeling that I couldn't get out. When I think of flying, I picture myself losing control, flipping out, and climbing the walls, but naturally I never ever did that. I m not afraid of crashing or hitting turbulence. It's just that sensation of being caught. Whenever I've thought of changing jobs, I've needed to believe, Would I be under pressure to fly? These days I only go places where I can drive or take a train. My good friends always point out that I couldn't leave a train taking a trip at high speeds either, so why don't trains bother me? I just tell them it isn't a reasonable worry.

A particular phobia is an intense, illogical worry of something that poses little or no real danger. Some of the more typical particular phobias are focused around closed-in places, heights, escalators, tunnels, highway driving, water, flying, pets, and injuries including blood. Such phobias aren't just severe worry; they are illogical worry of a specific thing. You might have the ability to ski the world's tallest mountains with ease but be not able to exceed the fifth floor of an office complex. While grownups with phobias realize that these fears are illogical, they often find that facing, or perhaps thinking about facing, the feared thing or circumstances brings on a panic attack or extreme anxiety.

Specific phobias affect an approximated 19.2 million adult Americans1 and are twice as typical in ladies as men.10 They normally appear in childhood or teenage years and tend to continue into the adult years.12 The reasons for specific phobias aren't well comprehended, but there is some proof that the tendency to develop them might run in families.

If the feared circumstances or feared thing is easy to stay away from, people with specific phobias may not seek assistance; but if avoidance disrupts their careers or their individual lives, it can become disabling and treatment is generally went after.
Specific phobias respond very well to thoroughly targeted psychotherapy.

A particular phobia includes being afraid of a particular circumstances or thing. When a specific experiences this, they tend to keep away from the item or area that they have a fear of.

The specific phobia is suffered by about a single person out of 10. It can be absolutely anything, but triggered by a specific object or circumstances. The fear is intense. In truth, it's a pan4ic attack. An example of the type of phobia consists of that of Arachnophobia, which is a fear of spiders.

Basic phobias might also be a fear of blood, medical interventions like injections, or injury. Victims might faint in the presence of blood or injury, following a decrease in their heart rate and blood pressure.

This is called a vasovagal reaction which causes fainting. It does not usually occur with other anxiety conditions. In other phobias and panic disorders the person's heart beat and blood pressure typically increases as their arousal rate boosts.

3. Spatial Fear (A non-specific) - A spatial phobia includes a particular location of the amount of space present. Agoraphobia is a typical phobia which can be defined as a generalized fear of leaving a familiar 'safe' place such as home, and of the possible panic attacks which may follow. It might also be a result of panic attack which in severe cases, avoids sufferers from leaving their homes unless joined by people they rely on. Agoraphobia is derived from a Greek word meaning "worry of the open marketplace".

Agoraphobia is different from panic attack, though lots of people who have panic attack typically suffer from agoraphobia. People who have panic attack go through repeating unforeseeable episodes of serious panic with no particular reason. Due to the intensity of symptoms which mark panic disorders, it is usually mistaken for lethal diseases such as a cardiac arrest. Signs consist of sweating, shortness of breath, hyperventilation, dizziness, unmanageable worry, quick heartbeat, and dizziness.

A non-specific phobia is a fear of a more generalized nature. Agoraphobia, for instance, is non-specific. The worry of open areas, or the more modern-day connected meaning where the worry includes remaining in a congested place.
What many non-sufferers find very tough to understand is that the phobia's fear is so usually of a non-threatening nature. I discussed buttons early on. Who in the world would be afraid of a button, we really wonder? The indicate understand, however, is that phobias have nothing whatever to do with the reasonable thinking part of the brain.
Understand, too, that the poor phobic can extremely typically see the irrationality of their fear themselves. It sounds just as silly to them too, but nevertheless whatever it may be still frightens them.

Some phobias talked about:

Acrophobia - Worry of Heights.

There is an important difference between fear of heights and acrophobia. I think we all have a particular worry of being up high. Worry is a mechanism for preservation. And there is definitely a threat when we find ourselves in a place where a slip in balance could lead us to putting ourselves at threat. So becoming afraid when in such a circumstance is a natural response of protection. It's when just the idea of being in an elevated place elicits an afraid or panicked reaction, then it's likely that you are handling a phobia.

Claustrophobia - Worry of Little Areas

There is a large series of reactions that have been categorized as claustrophobia. So if you start to feel a fear when you crawl into extremely little spaces where you are confined and would have trouble turning around that is one level of fear of small spaces. There is the other end of the spectrum where you feel panic when the door to your room is closed. Again the truly tight space fear can be thought about a regular response to be limited in movement. Again a conservation system, as we are programed with 2 responses to aggressive conduct. One way that we can react is by battling, and the other way is by running. I am sure you can see how being in a confined space would limit your ability to combat, and definitely eliminate your capability to run. So I do not think being in a really confined space is necessarily a phobic reaction, just a natural protective measure.

Nyctophobia - Worry of the Dark
This is a common worry in kids and may extend into adulthood. Just like the two preceding phobias, this is your own protective measure brought to an extreme. Among the primary ways in which we secure ourselves is through our senses. When we use our senses we can identify risk right before it is upon us and take action to ensure that we remain safe and alive. Among our primary senses that we have learned to trust is our sight. Darkness severely restricts our

capability to see things. There are animals that have exceptional capabilities to see in the dark, which puts us at a disadvantage when we are faced with that type of challenge.

The issue ends up being more worrisome when, because we can't see plainly, we begin to imagine some truly bad repercussions and we increase our worry response.

So as you can see, these three top phobias are truly regular fears that have been permitted to broaden and control our lives in undesirable and unwanted methods. One of the ways in which you can conquer your worries and phobias is with hypnosis and psychological images. When you take a look at the way these worries and phobias take place, you will see a typical link. They are all based upon our instinctual reaction of fight or flight, and our need to secure ourselves.

They are survival systems that are pre-programmed. The distinction between the phobia and the worry is the extent that you enable your creativity to take hold and magnify that worry to an illogical level with a trigger for instant reaction. When you use hypnosis you can learn to use your imagination more effectively.

A really good hypnotherapist can relieve you of the patterns that you have been practicing and help you to build correct mental imagery that will help you in staying calm and well balanced. It is indeed a widely known simple fact that a ton of individuals have particular kind of phobia, like worry for test or severe anxiety for public speaking.

Simply put, many of us experience a short duration of extreme worry as well as stress and anxiety in certain situations. In even worse cases, there are people who have prolonged phobias that put them under both psychological and physical distress for a prolonged period of time. Keep reading to discover the 3 main classifications of the phobias that are most frequently seen among us.

Brief summary of Phobias:

The fear of:
spiders (Arachnophobia).
social situations (social phobia).
flying (Aviatophobia).
open areas (Agoraphobia).
confined spaces (Claustrophobia).
heights (Acrophobia).
cancer (Cancerophobia).
thunderstorms (worry of lightening astraphobia; worry of thunder Brontophobia).
death (Necrophobia).
heart disease (Cardiophobia).

Another type of phobia which is very common nowadays is the agoraphobia. Bearing a certain degree of similarity to the formerly talked about social phobia, agoraphobia can be defined as the fear of open space. Typically, people who suffer from it would have anxiety attack too, since both signs are actually interconnected. Besides that, they will not be able to go to spots like shopping center, cinemas and so on as they will become panic.

The third category of phobia is simply pointing to the worry of a specific thing, animal, person or perhaps a particular situation. Truth to be told, this classification of phobia is the least severe among all the three classifications that we have discussed. People who suffer from this phobia will only experience anxiety condition when they enter into contact with that particular thing. Normally, this category of phobia is fairly much easier to deal with and many people have successfully overcame their worries through therapy and diagnosis.

Claustrophobia. Agoraphobia. Triskaidekaphobia.

All of these names have one thing in common: they include secret and confusion to what is already one of the most improperly understood aspects of human behavior.

Phobias have always been classified according to their obvious triggers; the items or situations that provoke the worry. These triggers are customarily dressed in exotic Greek and Latin labels, giving each phobia a more clinical air.

Symptoms of a Fear
All phobias can restrict your everyday activities and may cause serious anxiety and anxiety. Complex phobias, such as agoraphobia and social phobia, are most likely to cause these signs.

People with phobias usually intentionally stay away from entering contact with the thing that causes them fear and anxiety. For example, someone with a worry of spiders (arachnophobia) might not want to touch a spider and even look at an image of one.
In many cases, an individual can develop a real phobia where they become afraid of experiencing anxiety itself as it feels so awkward.

You don't have to be in the circumstances you're afraid of to experience the symptoms of phobia The brain is able to develop a response to terrifying circumstances even when you aren't actually in the situation.

The signs of a real phobia include experiencing extreme worry and anxiety when confronted with the situation or object that you are scared of. If your phobia is severe, thinking of the object of your phobia can also activate these signs. If you come near to, or into contact with, the feared circumstances you become anxious or distressed. In addition you may also have one or more undesirable physical symptoms.

An advancement of keeping away from the things of phobias is that this sort of behaviour can result in loss of Self-esteem which can in turn typically reinforce the fear related to the phobia. Frequently this can further turn into anxiety.
Signs of a phobia consist of:

Physical symptoms

People with phobias typically have panic attack. Anxiety attack can be very frightening and traumatic. The signs often happen unexpectedly and without caution.
As well as frustrating feelings of anxiety, a panic attack can trigger physical signs, like:
sweating
shivering
hot flushes or chills
shortness of breath or trouble breathing
a choking sensation
quick heartbeat (tachycardia).
strong pain or tightness in the chest.
an experience of butterflies in the stomach.
nausea.
headeache and lightheadedness.
feeling faint.
tingling or pins and needles.
dry mouth.
a need to go to the toilet.
sounding in your ears.
confusion or disorientation.
feeling unsteady, lightheaded, lightheaded or faint.
feeling like you are choking.
a pounding heart, palpitations or sped up heart rate.
chest pain or tightness in the chest.
hot or cold flushes.
shortness of breath or a smothering experience.
queasiness, vomiting or diarrhea.
tingling or tingling feelings.
trembling or shaking.

The physical signs are partly triggered by the brain which sends out a ton of messages down nerves to numerous parts of the body when you are restless. In addition, you launch tension hormonal agents - such as adrenaline (epinephrine) - into the blood stream when you are anxious. These can also act on the heart, muscles and other parts of the body to cause signs. You might even become anxious by just thinking of the feared situation. You wind up avoiding the feared situation as much as possible, which can limit your life and cause distress.

Mental symptoms.

In extreme cases, you might also experience psychological signs, such as:
fear of losing control.
fear of fainting.
feelings of fear.
fear of dying.
feeling out of touch with reality or detached from your body.

Experiencing this type of severe fear is extremely unpleasant and can be really frightening. It might make you feel stressed, out of control and overwhelmed. It might also lead to feelings of embarrassment, stress and anxiety or anxiety.

As a result, many people with phobias keep away from circumstances where they might have to face their worry. While this is an efficient technique to begin with, avoiding your worries often causes them to worsen, and can start to have a substantial impact on how you live your life.

The Very Best Treatment Methods
Various methods are said to deal with phobias. Their proposed advantages may vary from person to person.
Some therapists use virtual reality or images workout to desensitize clients to the feared entity. These belong to systematic desensitization therapy
Cognitive and behavior modifications help you to change certain ways that you think, feel and behave. They are useful treatments for numerous mental health issue, including phobias.

Cognitive treatment is based upon the idea that certain point of views can activate, or fuel, certain mental illness such as anxiety, anxiety and phobias. The therapist helps you to understand your present idea patterns. In specific, to determine any hazardous, unhelpful and false ideas or mindsets which you have that can make you anxious. The aim is then to change your ways of thinking to stay away from these ideas. Also, to help your thought patterns to be more sensible and helpful.

Behavioral therapy aims to change any behaviors which are harmful or not helpful. For instance, with phobias your response to the feared item (anxiety and avoidance) is not handy. The therapist helps you to change this. Various methods are used, depending upon the condition and situations. For example, for agoraphobia the therapist will normally help you to face up to feared circumstances, a little bit at a time. A first step may be to choose a really brief walk from your home with the therapist who gives support and guidance. In time, a longer walk may be possible, then a walk to the stores, then a trip on a bus, etc. The therapist might teach you how to manage stress and anxiety when you confront the feared circumstances and places. For example, by using deep breathing workouts. This strategy of behavior modification is called direct exposure therapy where you are exposed more and more to feared situations and learn how to cope.

Direct exposure treatment.
Because many phobic conditions include avoidance, direct exposure treatment, a particular psychotherapy, is the treatment of choice. With structure and assistance from a clinician who recommends exposure homework, clients seek out, challenge, and stay in contact with what they fear and stay away from until their anxiety is slowly relieved through a process called habituation. Since most clients know their fears are excessive and might be embarrassed by their fears, they are generally going to participate in this treatment ie, to keep away from staying away from.

Typically, clinicians start with a moderate direct exposure (eg, clients are asked to carefully approach the feared thing). If patients define velocity of their heart rate or shortness of breath when they encounter the feared circumstances or object, they may be taught to respond with sluggish, controlled breathing or other approaches that promote relaxation. Or, they might be asked to note when their heart rate sped up and shortness of breath began and when these response returned towards typical. When clients feel comfortable at one level of exposure, the direct exposure level is increased (eg, to touching the feared item).

Clinicians continue to increase the direct exposure level until patients can tolerate normal interaction with the circumstances or item (eg, ride in an elevator, cross a bridge). Exposure can increase as rapidly as clients endure it; often just a couple of sessions are needed.

Exposure treatment helps > 90% of patients who carry it out consistently and is almost always the only treatment needed for specific phobias.
Cognitive behavioral therapy (CBT) is a mix of the two where you may take advantage of changing both your thoughts and your conduct s.

CBT is generally done in weekly sessions of about 50 minutes each, for some weeks. You need to take an active part and are given research between sessions. For example, you might be asked to keep a journal of your thoughts which happen when you become restless.

Note: unlike other forms of talking treatments (psychiatric therapy), CBT does not look into the events of the past. CBT aims to handle your existing thought procedures and/or behaviors, and helps to change them where suitable. CBT typically works well to treat most phobias but doesn't suit everyone. Nevertheless, it might not be available on the NHS in all regions.

(CBT) can be helpful. Cognitive behavior modification allows the patient to challenge inefficient ideas or beliefs by bearing in mind their own emotions with the aim that the client will realize their fear is unreasonable. CBT may be conducted in a group setting. Gradual desensitization treatment and CBT are usually effective, offered the client is willing to endure some discomfort. In one medical trial, 90% of patients were observed with no longer having a phobic response after successful CBT treatment.

Antidepressant medications

These are frequently used to deal with anxiety. Nevertheless, they also help to decrease the signs of phobias (particularly agoraphobia and social phobia), even if you are not depressed. They work by interfering with brain chemicals (neurotransmitters) just like serotonin which may be associated with triggering stress and anxiety symptoms.

Antidepressants do not work straightaway. It takes 2 to 4 weeks right before their effect develops and anxiety is helped. A typical problem is that some people stop the medication after a week or so, as they feel that it is doing no good, and it is too early to tell if the medication is working.
Antidepressants are not tranquillizers and are not generally addicting.
There are some kinds of antidepressants, each with numerous benefits and drawbacks and they differ in their possible side-effects. However, selective serotonin reuptake inhibitor (SSRI) antidepressants are the ones most typically used for stress and anxiety and phobic disorders. Examples of SSRIs are citalopram and sertraline.
Note: after first beginning an antidepressant, in some people stress and anxiety symptoms can become worse for a few days right before they begin to improve. Your physician or practice nurse will want to keep an examine you in the very first weeks of treatment to see how you manage.
A combination of CBT and an SSRI antidepressant may work better in some cases than either treatment alone.

Benzodiazepines
Benzodiazepines such as diazepam are sometimes called small tranquilizers but they can have serious side-effects. They often work well in the short term to relieve symptoms of anxiety. The issue is they are addictive and can lose their effect if you take them for more than several weeks. They might also make you sleepy. Therefore, they are not a useful long-term treatment for phobias. A brief course, or even a single dosage, might be recommended for a phobia which happens hardly ever; however, there is no proof to support this practice. Recommendation for CBT or a fear of flying course (organized by a lot of airlines) is more efficient. Benzodiazepines may work in acute treatment of serious signs but the danger benefit ratio is really against their long term use in phobic disorders.
There are also new pharmacological techniques, which target learning and memory processes that happen throughout psychiatric therapy. For example, it has been shown that glucocorticoids can boost termination based psychotherapy.

Eye Movement Desensitization and Reprocessing
(EMDR) has been demonstrated in peer reviewed medical trials to be effective in treating some phobias. Mainly used to deal with Post traumatic stress condition, EMDR has been shown as effective in alleviating phobia signs following a specific trauma, such as a fear of pets following a dog bite Hypnotherapy combined with Eurolinguistics programs can also be used to help eliminate the associations that activate a phobic reaction.
However, lack of research and scientific testing jeopardizes its status as an efficient treatment.

Psychotherapeutic alternative medicine tool, also thought about to be pseudoscience by the mainstream medicine, is supposedly useful.

Another approach psychologists and psychiatrists use to deal with clients with severe phobias is extended direct exposure. Prolonged direct exposure is used in psychotherapy when the person with the phobia is exposed to the item of their fear over a long period of time. when an individual has overcome avoidance of or leave from the phobic item or situation. People with minor distress from their phobias usually do not need extended direct exposure to their worry.

These treatment choices aren't equally exclusive. Usually a therapist will suggest multiple treatments.

Efficient and Safe Herbal Remedies for Phobias
Whatever might be the reason there are effective natural treatments for phobia just like ginseng, lemon or lime, valerian root or lavender oil.
Lemon or Lime: The juice of a lemon or lime works for lowering lightheadedness or queasiness associated with a real phobia. Just cut a lemon into 2 halves and smell it for getting relief during an attack of phobia.
Ginseng: This herb is known for its stimulating and unwinding homes and is used thoroughly for the treatment of nerves.
Valerian Root: This herb can be used for the treatment of sleeping disorders. It has the homes for relaxing the nerves and the central nervous system of an agitated person and therefore is used as an efficient herbal remedy for the treatment of phobia. Grind 5-6 valerian roots for preparing the herbal remedy. It should be taken in 2-3 times a day for decreasing the impacts of phobia. However, pregnant and nursing mothers should stay away from the usage of the powder of valerian root.
Lavender: This is another reliable solution for phobia. Lavender has a soothing influence on the body and has an enjoyable odor. Daily lavender oil massage can help in eliminating an attack of phobia. The best way to lower stress is by including drops of lavender oil to the bathing water for a relaxing bath.
Kava: This is a well-known herb used for treating and sedating psychological clients. It relaxes the mind without hampering the mental clearness of the patients. Taking in the kava herb day-to-day builds up the tolerance level that is valuable in reducing phobia. The basic everyday dose of kava is 250 mg.
Passion Flower: The passion flower is a reliable natural extract that increases the performance of the nervous system and brain and helps to keep the organs in a healthy equilibrium. This natural treatment works in controlling phobias and panic.
Supragya Plus: In addition to the organic and natural remedies, there are certain ayurvedic solutions for phobia. Supragya plus is one such nerve tonic that strengthens the nerves and solves the nerve associated problems that consist of depression, stress and anxiety, phobia, stress, irritability, anger, intolerance, sleeplessness, palpitation and a lot more.
Ashwagandha: This is another efficient ayurvedic remedy that can be used in the treatment depression, stress and anxiety and other psychiatric conditions related with a phobia. The

leaves, roots, and berries of the herb have medical residential or commercial properties that prove to be effective in the treatment of an array of mental disorders.
Phobia is a serious mental disorder but with a healthy diet, correct workout and certain natural and ayurvedic treatments the issue can be successfully handled.

Getting rid of Phobias

While people might be amused by a good friend or family member shouting at the sight of a mouse or incapacitated with worry throughout a thunderstorm, phobias are no laughing matter for those whose lives are being adversely impacted. Fortunately, is that phobias are common and treatable and that comprehending a serious phobia is the primary step to overcoming it.

Fear is necessary to our survival. When we're scared, our primitive, automated fight or flight response is triggered. Afferent neuron fire in the brain and chemicals like adrenaline, noradrenaline and cortisol are released into our blood stream. In reaction, our breathing rate increases so we have trouble breathing. Blood is diverted from our digestive system to our limb muscles so our hearts pound and our stomachs churn. Our awareness intensifies. Our sight sharpens. Our impulses accelerate. We're now prepared to stand our ground and battle or run for our lives. Our forefathers needed this response to fight intruders or leave wild animals and it's just as essential today.

This reaction helps us make flash decisions to avert things like car accidents and sharpens our mental acuity so we can do things like meet abrupt due dates.

A fear has been referred to as a worry on steroids. For instance, it's regular to fear a snarling tiger. It's a real phobia, when you experience the same reaction fear when confronted by a friendly house cat.

Tackling phobias: what works?

There are many strategies to help get rid of phobias. Some you can try yourself and others need expert assistance. If your phobia is so severe that it sets off regular panic attacks and is negatively impacting your quality of your life, think about professional counselling.
Whether you're receiving professional aid or not, self-help strategies can make you feel more in control and that is the initial step to dominating any worry.

Here are several:

Relaxation methods.
Relaxation strategies such as deep breathing, meditation, and muscle relaxation are great ways to help you cope better with any stress and stress and anxiety in your life. With routine practice, they can enhance your ability to control the physical signs of anxiety, which will make facing your phobia less intimidating.

Challenging negative thoughts.
Altering distorted thinking patterns is part of what therapists call Cognitive Behavioral Therapy (CBT). The theory behind CBT is that our thinking (cognitive) affects the way we act (behavioral) and that by changing our thinking we can change our conduct. With phobias this requires determining and taking a look at negative beliefs that develop the distorted thought patterns that make us feel afraid.

These ideas are then challenged and changed with more realistic ones. For example, All pet dogs are vicious and will injure me. That idea is analyzed (what is the proof?) and challenged (that declaration is a gross overgeneralization) and ultimately changed with Not all canines are vicious. Most are kind and won't harm me.

Slowly facing your worries.
It makes sense to keep away from an object or situation that causes an intense and unpleasant response. However, that doesn't aid to conquer a serious phobia. Gradually facing your fear teaches your brain that your phobia might not be so frightening after all.
Many easy phobias can be effectively dealt with using a form of behavior modification referred to as exposure therapy or desensitization and can be finished with a therapist or without. It's done gradually. Each small step is repeated until the fear and stress and anxiety decreases. Only when you feel in control do you transfer to the next step.

For example, if you are scared of elevators, you may try the following steps:
1. Spend one minute in front of elevator doors.
2. Spend one minute checking out an elevator.
3. Spend one minute in an unmoving elevator with the door open.

For serious and complex concerns, desensitization treatment can take a considerable amount of time, but works well for less serious phobias.

There are also different medications available to help people deal with anxiety and these are usually used in conjunction with other treatments by medical occupations. So if your phobia continues to have an unfavorable influence on your life, connect for assistance. Phobias can be overcome often rapidly so there's no need to live your life in fear.

Interesting facts about phobias.
Phobias are more serious than simple fear experiences and are not restricted to fears of particular triggers.
Regardless of individuals knowing that their phobia is illogical, they cannot control the fear reaction.
Signs might include sweating, chest discomforts, and pins and needles.
Treatment can include medication and behavior modification.
Usually, particular phobias start in childhood, between 7 to eleven years with many cases starting before age 10.
Roughly 5% of kids and 16% of teenagers will have a specific phobia in their life time.
Girls are more likely to experience a serious phobia than boys at a rate of 2:1.
Fears are different than typical childhood worries. While kids normally become less scared of things like strangers, the bath, or the boogie beast, as they grow, kids with phobias usually become more scared as they mature. In addition, phobias hardly ever disappear by themselves. Phobias do not reduce with suitable reassurance and provision of info. For example, a dog phobia continues in spite of telling your child that grandmas dog is kind, has no teeth to bite because it is old, and will not scratch.

Some Reasons for a Phobia

Genetic and ecological factors can cause phobias. Children who have a close relative with a stress and anxiety condition are at threat of developing a phobia. Traumatic events, like almost drowning, can induce a serious phobia. Direct exposure to restricted spaces, severe heights, and animal or insect bites can all be sources of phobias.

People with ongoing medical conditions or health concerns usually have phobias. There's a high occurrence of people developing phobias after distressing brain injuries. Drug abuse and depression are also connected to phobias. Fears have different symptoms from serious mental illnesses such as schizophrenia. In schizophrenia, people have visual and acoustic hallucinations, deceptions, fear, negative signs like an hedonic, and disorganized signs. Fears may be irrational, but people with phobias do not fail reality screening.

A phobia is a fear, a worry that for many people is incapacitating and life changing. But let's just explore the entire concept of fear for a 2nd. Fear is great. Worry is a feeling that protects us when we are in risk. Think of a world without any worry, and you imagine a world of lawlessness and anarchy. Without fear, we would have little or no reward to behave and safeguard ourselves. Worry is our brain's way of safeguarding us.

Throughout the ages we have learned to be scared of certain things and situations. It is worry that secures us from snakes, sharks, and situations that can hurt us. We are right to be afraid of serpents-- lots of them are venomous and even if they don't kill us, we know that at finest we will feel pain. Similarly, we know that if we fall from a great height, the chances are we will break a leg or potentially die. So, in these circumstances we are right to feel fear, as it secures us.

Many people don't particularly like spiders or serpents, but they don't struggle with a major phobia. So when does a normal worry become a real phobia, and what causes some people to develop a real phobia of daily circumstances and things?

The answer to what causes a serious phobia is specific to each person, but certain circumstances may contribute to the circumstances. For instance, an individual who experiences a panic attack in an elevator might avoid taking an elevator after that for fear of experiencing another panic attack, in spite of the simple fact that the environment probably played no role in the initial
attack. The individual will, maybe unconsciously, blame the elevator for the attack, and ultimately the elevator and the anxiety attack ended up being so interlinked, that quickly a worry of elevators and confined areas has developed, and the individual now suffers from claustrophobia.

A serious phobia may also be inherited, or rather taught. Take the case of Brian, an 11yr old boy who is afraid of flying. Why is an 11yr old so scared of flying? The answer might be that his mother is also scared. We learn much from our mother and father, and trust them to protect us. Therefore, if our parent, who is supposed to protect us, is scared of something, we learn that it must be damaging and that we too should hesitate of it. The huge risk here is that what may be a moderate fear in a moms and dad, can turn into a full incapacitating phobia in a child.

The just one thing that all phobias have in common is that they are psychological, and for that reason the treatment of phobias lies there. By understanding why we experience a particular phobia, we can begin to treat it. One of the best ways of dealing with phobias is with hypnosis. Hypnosis works by re-training the mind subconsciously to react to the phobia in a different way. By doing it subconsciously, a great deal of the stress and stress and anxiety is taken out of the treatment for the client-- for lots of people, even speaking about their phobia can cause extreme stress.

Just one thing that everybody who conquers their phobia has in common is a big sense of relief. When we face up to, and overcome our worries we begin to realize how we have been held back, and the enormous sense of liberty is overwhelming. That doesn't mean that phobias can be considered minor or banal-- they're far from it. For sufferers, they are very real, and all consuming. At http://www.free-hypnosisdownloads.com there is a growing number of outstanding hypnosis mp3 downloads that help victims of various kinds of phobias to conquer them easily and quickly. The download sessions usually last about 30-40mins to listen to, and their success rate is rather incredible.

Hypnosis is so effective in the treatment of phobias since it addresses the phobia in precisely the same way that it got there in the first place-- subconsciously. This makes the entire experience so much more satisfying for the topic, and for that reason the likelihood of success is incredibly high.

Social Phobias

When an individual is extremely awkward and also has severe amounts of anxiety concerning social situations, it is called social stress and anxiety. It is also described as social phobia and is a disorder. These people constantly have the fear of being judged, watched or slammed. These people have such a great amount of worry that it does disrupt life at school, work, and any kind of social activity or perhaps with everyday life. The majority of these people do understand that the fear is something that is not actually needed but are still not able to stop it.

Social phobia is also one form of phobia. A few people feel afraid to drink or even eat in front of other individuals. Some of them do not speak in front of other people also. Some of the cases may be so extreme that the person is terrified to speak to another person. Physical symptoms develop in a lot of the cases of social phobia. They include blushing, sweating, talking with problem, palpitations, trembling, discomfort in the stomach and many more. It makes it very basic if they deal with these issues rather than fretting more about it.

Social phobia might be triggered because of many a reason. In might be just because of the simple fact that it runs in the family. Therefore, the children get the exact same problems from their mom and dad. It may also be due to alcoholism or due to depression. In women social depression happens two times as much as men for reasons which we do not know. It may start at youth or perhaps at adolescence. It hardly ever begins at 25 years of age. Researches have been going on in this field to learn all the problems that are causing social phobia.

Some of the researchers have been blaming the cause if these signs on a small structure present in the brain which is called amygdale. Our sense of worry is what is controlled by this amygdale. Another group of scientists really believe that this social phobia is passed down from generation to generation.

Yet another group of researchers say that the reason for this social phobia is because of a sensitivity that is very high to disapproval, it may also be based upon physiological reasons or on hormones.

The environment may be yet another reason for the reason for social phobia according to a few researchers. This may be because of something that happened to another person in the same situation. It is called observational learning. This simply put is learning to behave based upon others around you.

Environmental and genetic elements result in phobias. Kids who are prone to anxiety conditions are at a higher danger of developing these phobias. Extreme heights, restricted areas, exposure to insect or animal bites or an upsetting event like near drowning could be a source of such phobias. Even those people with chronic medical conditions just like drug abuse, anxiety or brain injuries are prone to developing these phobias.

Throughout the last few decades, scientists, psychologists and doctors have investigated and analyzed lots of people who struggle with different kinds of Phobia. The very first thing to keep in mind here is once more that Phobias are incredibly complex and there is no chance to tell with 100% certainty that someone is experiencing a phobia.
Phobias-banner-zafirides2

However, there are clear signs that most of phobias develop throughout early childhood, teenage years or early adulthood. It is rather unusual for a serious phobia to develop out of absolutely nowhere after the age of 30 35. Phobias can be brought on by difficult circumstances, certain experiences or frightening events. It is also understood that kids can develop the same phobia among their parents struggled with if they were progressively aware of this during childhood.

Causes for the Simple Phobias

Specific (or simple) phobias often appear to develop in early childhood between the ages of 4 and 8 years of age. Certain events in life or unpleasant experiences can usually plant a seed, which will grow overtime and slowly develop into some sort of phobia. For instance, an undesirable experience in a confined (or small) space could possibly cause claustrophobia in a later stage of life.

Doctors have found that phobias aren't always genetically acquired from either of the mom and dad. However, if a child is progressively aware of one of its father and mother phobia, chances are much higher that this child will develop the exact same (or a similar) phobia during later phases in life. For instance, if a mother experiences Arachnophobia (worry of spiders) then it is far more very likely for her daughter to develop the exact same phobia as well, simply since she was highly aware of her mom's fear throughout childhood.

Causes for Complex Phobias

Like the name suggests, the causes for complex and/or social phobias are still shrouded in clouds of mystery and uncertainty. Scientists believe that the complex phobias are typically triggered by a combination of genetics, brain chemistry and certain life experiences. It is said that social phobias are more likely to be brought on by a very demanding experience than agoraphobia.
Some say that there may be an evolutionary clarification for some kinds of phobias. In age-old times for example, staying outdoors in a wide and open field would increase the risk of getting caught by other unsafe predators. For that reason, it's only logical that for lots of people, specifically for young children, there is a strong instinct for staying safe in the house.

Furthermore, today's social phobias could have been a potential survival instinct in old times. Staying with a group of complete strangers (people from another tribe perhaps) was far more hazardous countless years ago than it is now. Very few people today in a congested mall will want to battle you over your newly caught deer.

Another highly acceptable cause for complicated phobias might be found in the field of neuroscience. Some areas of the brain (see image) are understood to store info about dangerous and even fatal events. If a similar event is faced at some point in the future, the brain will automatically recall those old memories and make the body react as if it were a recurrence. As phobias are irrational phenomena, in some cases it's possible to deal with victims by managing to get the brain to change the bad and negative memories of certain events with something more rational and rational. Nevertheless, the parts of the brain that handle worry typically keep recovering the bad memories. This makes it very difficult to find an extremely effective medical treatment for complicated phobias.

Much is still unidentified about the real reason for some phobias. Causes may also include:

Tons of phobias develop as a result of having a negative experience or panic attack related to a specific thing or situation.

There may be a link between your own specific phobia and the phobia or stress and anxiety of your father and mother this could be as a result of genetics or learned behavior.

Changes in brain working also may play a role in developing particular phobias.

Danger elements
These aspects might increase your threat of particular phobias:

Your age.
Particular phobias can first appear in childhood, usually by age 10, but can occur later in life.

Your relatives.
If somebody in your family has a specific phobia or anxiety, you're more likely to develop it, too.
This could be an acquired propensity, or kids might learn particular phobias by observing a
family member's phobic response to a things or a scenario.

Your temperament.
Your threat may increase if you're more sensitive, more hindered or more negative than the
norm.

An unfavorable experience.
Experiencing a frightening terrible event, such as being trapped in an elevator or attacked by an
animal, might set off the development of a specific phobia.

Finding out about negative experiences.
Hearing about negative information or experiences, such as airplane crashes, can result in the
development of a particular phobia.

Problems

Although specific phobias may appear ridiculous to other ones, they can be devastating to the
people who have them, triggering issues that impact many aspects of life.

Social isolation. Staying away from spots and things you fear can trigger academic, professional
and relationship problems. Children with these disorders are at threat of scholastic issues and
solitude, and they might have trouble with social skills if their habits considerably differ from
their peers.
Mood conditions. Many people with particular phobias have depression in addition to other
stress and anxiety disorders.
Substance abuse. The tension of living with an extreme particular phobia may cause abuse of
drugs or alcohol.
Suicide. Some people with specific phobias may be at danger of suicide.

Environmental and hereditary elements lead to phobias. Kids who are vulnerable to anxiety
disorders are at a greater danger of developing these phobias. Extreme heights, confined
spaces, direct exposure to insect or animal bites or a distressing event like near drowning could
be a source of such phobias. Even those people with persistent medical conditions like
substance abuse, depression or brain injuries are susceptible to developing these phobias.

It is uncommon for a phobia to begin after the age of 30 years, and the majority of start throughout early youth, the teenage years, or early their adult years.

They can be caused by a demanding experience, a frightening event, or a moms and dad or household member with a real phobia that a kid can 'learn.'

There doesn't seem to be one particular reason for phobias, but there are some factors that might play a crucial role:

Specific incidents or injuries. For example, somebody who experiences a ton of turbulence on an aircraft at a young age may later develop a serious phobia about flying.
Learned responses, picked up in early life. Factors in the family environment, such as parents who are very anxious or restless, can have an impact on the way you manage anxiety in later life. You might develop the exact same particular phobia as a parent or older sibling.
Genetics. Some research suggests that some people are more susceptible to developing a phobia than others.
Reactions to stress or fear. If you have a strong response (or panic attack) in response to a specific situation or object, and you find this humiliating or people around you react strongly, it can trigger you to develop more intense stress and anxiety about being in that situation again. Long-term stress can cause emotions of anxiety and depression and minimize your ability to cope in specific circumstances. This can make you feel more afraid or restless about being in those situations again and, over a long period, could lead to you developing a serious phobia.

Social and particular phobias in some cases run in families, providing proof of a genetic connection. Some people are born with a predisposition towards stress and anxiety, which makes them especially susceptible to developing phobias.

Phobias might develop as a reaction to pressure or following terrible events. In other cases, unreasonable fears might develop with no evident trigger. Adults usually recognize that their worries are unreasonable or excessive, and this can serve as a separating factor. The impacted person may not speak with friends and family about a fear that they actually believe is ridiculous.

Phobias are also a natural part of development. A lot of kids go through phases where they are scared of the dark, of monsters, or of strangers. A lot of teens develop stress and anxieties associated with self-image and other ones' understanding of them.

While these fears are normal and often get left behind gradually, they can sometimes persist or become incapacitating.

Everybody has things that terrify them. Nevertheless, there are some people who have strong, irrational, and involuntary responses to everyday things and places, which are called phobias.

There have been some studies examining the causes of phobias, but there is still no real consensus regarding why some people have this type of reaction to certain stimuli. Fears are probably more typical than you may believe according to the National Institutes of Mental Health and the American Psychiatric Association, about 7 to 9 percent of adults in the United States struggle with a particular phobia.

Twenty-one percent of those adults suffer from serious phobias, which translates to about 2 percent of the entire population. Many phobias can be linked to a particular event or situation in the formative years of childhood, but it's not always clear what triggers these phobias.

In most cases, specific phobias develop in early youth between the ages of 7 and 11, though it is possible for a phobia to develop at any age. Particular phobias can be brought on by a variety of different aspects: experiencing a distressing event (e.g. being attacked by a pet dog); observing other ones going through a distressing event (e.g. witnessing a car accident); an unforeseen anxiety attack (e.g. while flying in an airplane); or informative transmittal (e.g. substantial media coverage of a terrorist attack).

Usually, those affected by a specific phobia are not able to identify the reason why their phobia developed. While the cause of a particular phobia may be unidentified, it is necessary to recognize the symptoms and remember that phobias can be treatable if you look for aid from a mental health specialist.

Chapter 7: Tourette's Syndrome

Tourette syndrome, aka Gilles de la Tourette syndrome, is a neurological or neurochemical disorder that can be characterized by tics. Tics are involuntary, fast, abrupt motions or vocalizations that happen repeatedly in the same way. Symptoms to Tourette's consist of several motor and many times some singing tics present at a long time during the disorder. These different tics aren't required to take place simultaneously.

The event of tics throughout the day usually happens is spasms. These convulsions happen nearly every day or intermittently throughout a period of more than one year. The syndrome will change in the amount, frequency, type and place of the affecting tics.

Vocal tics can be partitioned into different categories, including:

- Repetition of words after reading them

- Spontaneous utterance of socially questionable words (Normally Racial and ethnic).

- Repeating of one's own formerly spoken words.

- Repetition of words spoken by someone else after being heard by the person with the condition.

Besides the singing tics, there are lots of other classifications which do not always included word repetition. Tourette syndrome singing tics do not even need to be words; they can be represented by almost any possible brief vocal noise. The most typical of these kinds of tics are noises produced that look like throat cleaning, short cough, grunts, or moans.

Motor tics can be a countless variety of actions which can include:

- Bent facial grimacing.

- Knuckles banging together.

- Itching.

- Hand-clapping.

- Scratching.

Tourette's Syndrome is indicated when a person exhibits both multiple motor and one or more singing tics over the period of 1 year, without any more than three months of consecutive living tic-free. These Tic disturbances can easily impair and or distress the person from working normally. The diagnosis cannot be involved with drug abuse or another medical condition, and should be before the age of 18.

History of the Syndrome

Tourette syndrome is a brain condition in which the affected person has multiple tics both physical and spoken. The disorder affects more than one hundred thousand Americans. There has been written evidence of Tourette syndrome since at least the 15th Century. The Jakob Sprenger and Heinrich Kraemer book Malleus Maleficarum ("Witch's Hammer"), which was published in 1489, defined a priest with unusual tics.

Throughout the 19th century, the formal recognition and naming of the disorder took place. In 1825, French physician, Jean Gasparted Itard, detailed the case of Marquise de Dampierre, lady of nobility, who experienced episodes of coprolalia. Madam Dampierre, who otherwise had improved good manners fitting of her social standing and education, would make vulgar statements showing weird conduct.

In the 1880s, prominent French physician Jean-Martin Charcot was interested in studying the condition. In 1885, his protégé, Georges Gilles de la Tourette, a French neurologist, released a report of nine clients with the condition. The particular goal of the research studies was to define a disease range from chorea and hysteria. Tourette studied psychotherapy, hypnosis, and hysteria as part of his work.

Tourette's released report "maladie des tics" concluded by specifying that a new scientific classification needed to be defined for the disorder. Charcot consequently named the condition in Tourette's honor.

Tourette syndrome was initially thought to be a psychological condition. However, this view has changed since research throughout the 1970s. This brand-new research supported that the condition has a neurological cause. More just recently, a view that integrates biological predisposition with environmental elements has been more widely accepted. However, there is still no clear consensus as how to finest classify the condition.

Tourette syndrome affects people worldwide. Cases have been reported in more than 50 countries varying from Australia to Brazil, Poland to China, and Turkey to South Africa. Since the condition is usually not diagnosed as Tourette syndrome or medical treatment is not looked for, it is challenging to determine how many people experience the disorder.

Some Typical Causes

The causes of Tourette syndrome have yet to be established even though people have suffered with the condition for centuries. However, evidence does show that the condition roots from abnormal activity in a neurotransmitter called dopamine. Other neurotransmitters, like serotonin, might be involved as well. Genes seems to play a part in the condition, so it also appears to be inherited. Whether the individual is male or female affects the display of the gene.

If one moms and dad has the condition, there is a half chance that a kid will acquire it. Acquiring the disorder is three times higher for a son than it is for a child. Emotional and physical health or external tension also adds to the development of the condition. Tics present more when one with the disorder undergoes stress, unnecessary pressure or severe tiredness. An inner sensation that is awkward is relieved through the tic process.

Noradrenaline is said to be the most considerable promote that triggers the different tics as medications that imitate noadrenaline triggers the uncontrolled behavior. Some people with underlying brain conditions that are inherited from birth can get this condition. But the majority of people with Tourette do not have another underlying condition. Also, people who have had brain infections, just like meningitis, have movements extremely comparable to tics once they recover. But this is unusual. Research is still being performed on the causes of Tourette syndrome and there is hope that a remedy will be found in the future.

Did you know that Tourette's syndrome affects over 200,000 Americans in the United States? Signs normally commence in youth and luckily, aren't degenerative in nature. Pharmacological medications have progressed that help limit and even entirely reduce symptoms thanks to brand-new innovative advances. TS signs might reduce or diminish during sleep, but rarely entirely disappear which can make sleeping tough sometimes.

The newest kinds of treatment methods include looking into the genetic basis for Tourette s. Researchers have discovered based on twin and family research studies that TS is indeed acquired. Recent research has yielded intriguing findings as well. Previous info sited that those with Tourette's need to only get among the malfunctioning genes to exhibit symptoms and signs of TS. Specialists now really believe that ecological elements and minor chromosomal differences result in the development of full-blown and even moderate cases of Tourette's syndrome. Some individuals might be providers for TS, but not develop the condition at all based upon complicated hereditary combinations.

Genetically speaking, gender also effects how Tourettes Syndrome is uttered. Women tend to manifest more obsessive-compulsive signs like recurring habits (counting, washing, ordering, and setting up) whereas male patients are much more very likely to have motor tics or abrupt, quick, recurring movements involving a specific, minimal group of muscles within the body. These tics may even be vocal in form.

By examining hereditary precursors and expressions researchers are better able to use genetic therapy to identify and advise members of the family in sees to treatment choices and even restorative techniques to help with issues such as sleep disruption. As research advances in the field of Tourettes treatment we can expect to see further developments and quality of life improvements for those managing TS.

Diagnosing It

There is no simple test to detect this condition. Blood tests, EKGs and other ones are essentially worthless when trying to identify whether a client has Tourette syndrome. The best way to reach an accurate scientific medical diagnosis is to have your health history and signs evaluated by a skilled doctor. Once a medical diagnosis has been acquired, there are some treatment techniques that can be used to help ease the signs. Researchers and scientists have no information on what triggers Tourette's.

Research studies have shown that this can be an inherited disease which means that it can be passed from parents on to their children but more studies are needed so as to identify the specific cause of the illness and any possible way to prevent it in those who are inclined. One thing that you can do is to learn as much as you can about the condition. It often helps to read stories by others who have been detected. Often understanding that you are not alone is the best treatment. Tourette's by Chris Mason is often advised by medical professionals whose patients suffer from Tourette syndrome. This book includes letters from parents of children with the disease in addition to grownups who have been detected. It gives you an idea of the troubles that others have faced attempting to come up with the appropriate medical diagnosis and helps those with Tourette's to feel a bit less alone.

Some Typical Realities

One of the essential truths about Tourette Syndrome is that it is acquired. This is a neural disorder that triggers involuntary motions also referred to as tics. The onsets of these movements are normally facial tics like blinking of the eyes or nose twitches. With time, though, other symptoms may present which can include head jerking or foot stomping.

People with Tourette syndrome, also referred to as TS, may also involuntarily shout out obscene words or odd expressions. It has been known that people with serious TS can be damaging to themselves by head banging or biting. Tics happen more when the person is in a stressful circumstances and less typically when they are relaxed. TS patients can often control their Tics to a particular degree, but eventually the conduct might finally appear worse after trying to restrain it.

The typical beginning of TS happens between the ages of 7-10 and can happen to any ethnic group. It is not known why as of yet, but it appears to impact males 3-4 times more often than it does females. There is no treatment for TS and because it doesn't impair most clients, no medication is really needed. If it does hinder a patient's ability to function, a type of Neuroleptics may be recommended.

There is no medicine that can suppress all the numerous tics from which an individual might suffer and some of these medications have side effects that are far worse than the tics themselves. Most kids with Tourette syndrome can function just fine in a typical classroom but if the tics get regrettable, it may be best to put them in a special class or school that can help them excel. Some physicians might refer a person with TS to a therapist just to help the client learn better how to deal with life and reduce stress.

More Symptoms

People with Tourette's experience tics, which are body language or sounds that occur unpredictably and periodically.

An individual with Tourette's may exhibit regular behavior the vast majority of the time. Nevertheless, the beginning and amount of tics displayed is unpredictable and the amount varies. Some days a person with Tourette's might experience a multitude of tics while the next day, they might experience just a few.

To be diagnosed with Tourette's the person should experience both motor and singing tics for a prolonged time period. Shoulder shrugging, facial grimacing, eye blinking, and head jerking are motor tics. Examples of singing tics would include sniffing, throat clearing, yelping, tongue clicking, and other sounds.

Two of the most typical tics for people with Tourette's are throat clearing and eye blinking. Other tics people with Tourette's experience include facial movements, coughing, humming, smelling, grunting, and shoulder shrugging. Fixations, compulsions, impulsivity, negligence, and state of mind irregularity can also be characteristics of the condition.

Tourette's is the most serious of spectrum of tic disorders. There are two classifications of tics, basic and complex. Example of more complex motor tics would be smelling, leaping, touching other people or things, twirling about, or more seldom self-injurious actions like hitting one's own head as biting oneself. More complex singing tics are using socially inappropriate words in public or saying words or phrases out of context. This is referred to as coprolalia.

Coprolalia is the frequently associated sign of Tourette's as it is regularly used in showing people with the condition in movies, television, and other kinds of media. Other symptoms of Tourette's include echolalia, which is the repeating the words of other individuals, and palilalia, which is repeating one own words.

With Tourette's, the tics can come all of a sudden and vary in type. However, the tics connected with the condition are temporarily suppressible, in contrast to other movement disorders. This appears in the simple fact that older kids and grownups are far better able to manage their tics than younger children, when Tourette's syndrome signs are normally most noticable.

Sociological and Cultural Aspects of Tourette's Syndrome

More than 50% of the population doesn't acknowledge Tourette's.
Tourette Syndrome is specified as a neural disorder which triggers uncontrolled motions, consisting of facial twitches, blinking, shrugging, nodding, stomping, and a wide variety of other movements (in some rare cases people have behaviors that are socially inappropriate).

Periodically it involves uncontrolled noises, just like chirping, sniffing, grunting, whistling, barking, and in extremely extreme cases, shouting and even swearing.

Sociological and Cultural Elements of TS
When people notices you twitching and making unusual noises occasionally, they would typically ask you to stop doing it or try to repeat the exact same action that you just did inadvertently, leaving you in absolutely embarrassed. Or in many cases, they would give you nicknames just like twitchy and tease you.

Many people tend to pushes away Tourette's victims and presume that they are psychologically challenged. In truth, people with Tourette's can be just as clever as anybody who doesn't have Tourette's.

Understand and Acknowledge TS
1) Some Tourette's syndrome is genetic.
2) Tourette's is absolutely not infectious.
3) Tourette's does not equate to being psychologically challenged. They are typical people with just a few motor specials needs.
4) Tourette's victims are refraining from doing those actions or noises deliberately, they are mostly unmanageable. Just like how you can't keep back a yawn or a sneeze.

Tics and Tourette's Syndrome in Kids

The symptoms of tics and Tourette's syndrome normally manifest themselves between the ages of three and ten years old and consist of unchecked, repetitive, fast movements that take place involuntarily for no evident reason. More typical tic motions include eye blinking and throat clearing; these often happen when the person is stressed out, tired, anxious, or under the impact of certain medications. Both motions and noises may be repeated, in some cases all at once, but often exclusively. Those with tic or Tourette's syndrome usually have their most apparent signs between the ages of 9 and 13. Over half improve throughout their teen years and into early their adult years; however, some have moderate to severe tics into the adult years. In some cases specific tics go away while other ones stay.

Tourette's syndrome is an acquired neuropsychiatric disorder. Its most typically associated with verbal tics that involve the sudden shouting of obscene remarks; nevertheless, not all tics are verbal. Other tics can be physical - like fidgeting with hair or unbuttoning outfits. Eye blinking, coughing, sniffing and facial motions are also common. Some tics are unnoticeable to others, like toe crunching or abdominal flexing. Between one and 10 kids per 1,000 have Tourette's, which is the term used for a spectrum of tic conditions. Tic conditions have nothing to do with a kid's intelligence, life expectancy or levels of individual health. The precise cause of the syndrome is unidentified.

Tics alone aren't damaging, but the can definitely impact your kid's daily life. Because of this, you may want to seek treatment to keep the tics under control. There are medications available to lower signs, but they typically have adverse effects of their own, and regrettably there is no single medication to eradicate all symptoms entirely. In many cases, doctors and families choose to pass up medication and focus rather than managing the environmental elements that can add to the manifestation of tics, which usually fluctuate in severity, depending on a number of elements. As there is no universal prescription to deal with tic disorders, passing up medication entirely stays away from needing to try different types of medicinal interference which can usually have negative effects more troubling than symptoms for which they were recommended. The majority of treatment involves creating a supportive environment for the child. It's also important for the kid to learn relaxation methods to stay away from tension, which can activate the tics. Relaxation training, yoga, meditation and exercise have been found to help in some cases.

Among the most important aspects of these conditions to consider is the simple fact that your kid has no control over the recurring tics or motions. Trying to stop them or talk them into soothing down will not work and can only trigger more tension and anxiety. It's also crucial to clarify this to teachers and other school officials who will come into contact with your child. Focusing way too much on the tics can make the signs worse. Creating a system of loving assistance can be more efficient than any prescription - and such a system generally involves more people than just the mother and father.

Handling Tics in your home and at School

Tourette syndrome or TS is a genetic, Neuro-chemical disorder defined by uncontrolled muscle movement called tics. These tics can look like simple repetitive motions like blinking or exaggerated actions like gyrations on the floor.

Working with kids with TS can be difficult particularly when they in some cases present with accompanying conditions such as ADHD and OCD (Compulsive Compulsive Condition). Rage or aggressive conduct has been reported as a clinical issue in about 25-40% of TS clients. Nevertheless, understanding the mechanics behind the syndrome can bring about effective management of the Tourette syndrome kid in the class.

What is a Tic?
Incorporating the TS kid into a regular classroom works best when the kids in the class comprehend what a tic is. Tics often begin as awkward tingling advises or feelings to move a set of muscles. Research studies suggest that repressing a tic is not a really good idea since the urge becomes increasingly insistent until it ends up being an outburst. Telling the children in class what a tic is and highlighting how it is as natural as sneezing can teach them the importance of sympathy and understanding for those who are different. Too, this technique de-mystifies the syndrome. A tic is as natural to the TS child as a sneeze. Additionally, tics typically disappear in frequency and seriousness as the child grows older. They are hardly noticeable after the age of 19.

This being said, it is worthy to keep in mind that lots of instructors claim that tics can be just stopped in mid-track through diversion or distraction. Motivating the Tourette syndrome child to focus on a set of mathematics problems or checking out a book can actually divert his attention from the tic and cool down the involuntary muscle motions. One teacher claims that her TS child gets on the computer when she feels a tic coming one. Physically moving the mouse and concentrating on the screen are enough to stop the approaching tic.

Moms And Dad Management Training
Parent management training has an effective impact on the disruptive behavior of kids with TS. This training can help with explosive outbursts in the home.
In a 2006 research study, one group of mom and dad was taught 3 primary strategies for conduct management:
a) Consistency in their reactions to blasts and outbursts
b) Clearness in clarification of consequences
c) Choice of positive, instead of negative, repercussions.
A 2nd group of father and mother got no training whatsoever. Results arranged at the end of the 10 week study showed that the trained mom and dad reported 32% less disruptive occurrences than the un-trained mother and father.

Cognitive Behavior Modification
If moms and dad management training is not practical, families can turn to cognitive behavior modification, a form of training that works on the assumption that habitual behavioral reactions can be modified by changing idea patterns. Dealing with professionally trained therapists, the Tourette syndrome kid can learn to identify unsuitable expressions of feelings. They also learn to substitute a much different conduct or diversion (such as reading or painting) for these situations. With practice and perseverance, many TS children learn to break their old pattern of anger and hostility by turning to more acceptable and positive reactions.

The Tourette syndrome kid can be a favorable enhancement in a regular class. His or her interaction with other kids is a good chance for developing sympathy, understanding and behavior management for all.

Dieting

Many nutritionists believe that Tourettes and diet can be connected together to help people who suffer from this disorder. Tourettes Syndrome is a neural condition that causes outbursts that are absolutely uncontrollable. These outbursts are called "tics." Tics are movements or sounds that are recurring and completely involuntary. Nearly 200,000 Americans have this condition and a lot of cases are rather severe. Many healthcare specialists believe that a diet including anti-yeast foods and the yeast fighter, Nystatin, can truly help patients.

Tourettes syndrome appears to be exceptionally sensitive to yeast. The intestinal tracts take in the yeast, which is frequently found in bread. Acetone, which is a by-product of yeast, has been found to slow down the processes of the brain. Yeasts are really conscious Nystatin, which is an anti-fungal drug and can be used with a diet plan including no yeast. Tics are related to the lack of Magnesium in the diet as well. It is incredibly essential to include Magnesium to the diet for proper nerve and muscle function.

Foods that are high in Magnesium are some seafood, green veggies, beans, nuts, bananas, and tofu. Magnesium pills can also be taken to help enrich the diet. A medical trial is presently being performed at John's Hopkins University. In the trial, physicians are putting clients on a customized Atkins diet. This diet manages how much sugar and carbs are in the diet. By doing this, Ketosis can begin to develop in the body. Ketosis helps the body use less fat for energy. Hopefully, research trials just like this will supply better ways to treat Tourettes and provide a better quality of life for clients who experience TS.

Natural Treatments

Tourette Syndrome (TS) is usually plant other disorders, like attention deficit/hyperactivity disorder (ADHD) and obsessive/compulsive condition (OCD). TS and OCD have actually been genetically linked, but both aren't always present. It is believed that OCD and ADHD can develop or worsen because of the presence of Tourette Syndrome. People familiar with their tics generally become obsessed with managing them and find it extremely hard to sit still or take note.

Tests can be done to see if there are physiological reasons for the tics to manifest. Tests usually are ordered to check for seizures and hypothyroidism. TS is usually misdiagnosed as autism just because of the resemblance of behaviors.

Parents of children identified with Tourette Syndrome can be desperate to find assistance. This is specifically real because ADHD and OCD signs can be really debilitative in a school setting. Children with Tourette Syndrome typically have major trouble focusing, managing outbursts, remaining on job and writing.

Tics can usually be managed for an extended amount of time, similar to refusing to scratch an itch. But, ultimately a giant outburst must take place and the itch must be scratched. Parents of kids with Tourette Syndrome that report etiquette at school usually have a dreadful time at home with behavior, stress and anxiety, control and opposition.

People with tics typically do finest if they are in a helpful environment. The perception of the seriousness of tics seems to be far more essential for development than the actual severity of tics. There are no medical treatments for Tourette Syndrome that do not have adverse negative effects, so behavioral, mental and cognitive treatments are more advantageous in most cases.

Dealing with Tourette Syndrome naturally is just something that lots of mom and dad are looking into. The tics and symptoms can come and go, so it may be tough to tell if your treatment is working as planned. Furthermore, symptoms can worsen all the way approximately age 12 and can perhaps get a lot better through teenage years. Many adults still have very mild tics, but many don't even see them.

So if your child is young and you are dealing with symptoms, you might be backward and forward between thinking that it is really working and thinking that it is not working at all, but it could just be the natural progression of the condition. You could be helping a lot more than you know, even when symptoms continue to worsen.

Dealing with TS habits and signs with vitamins and supplements can be a natural way to help your child lessen the trauma, anxiety and anxiety that can take place because of the tension and unwanted behaviors brought on by TS. You can regulate stress and anxiety and tension causing hormonal agent cortisol by taking vitamins E, B and C. You can decrease neurosensitivity by supplementing with DHA fish oils. A lot of children and adults with Tourette Syndrome are deficient in vitamin C, which is responsible for keeping serotonin levels in check. You might want to supplement with vitamin C powder to get a high enough dosage of vitamin C to be effective. As always, talk with your physician before starting a vitamins and supplement programs.

Ayurvedic Treatments

The Ayurvedic treatment of TS is targeted at managing the tics and stopping neurobehavioral complications. Medicines like Yograj-Guggulu, Maha-Rasnadi-Guggulu, Maha-Vat-Vidhwans-Ras, Vat-Gajankush-Ras and Dashmoolarishta are used to manage the involuntary motions. Organic medicines which can be used in this condition consist of Shallaki (Boswellia serrata), Guggulu (Commiphora mukul), Rasna (Pluchea lanceolata), Tagar (Valeriana wallichii), Deodar (Cedrus deodara), Erandmool (Ricinus communis), Chitrak (Plumbago zeylanica), Vishwa (Zinziber officinalis), Shalparni (Desmodium gangeticum), Prushnaparni (Uraria picta), Agnimanth (Premna mucronata) and Shyonak (Oroxylum indicum).

People who do not respond to the above discussed treatment can be given other medicines like Ekang-Veer-Ras, Tapyadi-Loh, Kaishor-Guggulu, Trayodashang-Guggulu, Vish-Tinduk-Vati and Bruhat-Vat-Chintamani. Sedative herbs like Sarpagandha (Rauwolfia serpentina), Jatamansi (Nardostachys jatamansi), Khurasani ova (Hyoscyamus niger) and Jaiphal (Myristica fragrans) also help in giving relief from tics. Medicated oils like Mahanarayan oil, Mahamash oil, Chandan-Bala-Laxadi oil, Vishgarbha oil and Maha-Saindhavadi oil are applied in your area. This is followed by localized steam fomentation of the afflicted parts using medications like Nirgundi-Qadha and Dashmool-Qadha.

Since TS is usually associated with other neurobehavioral issues, extra medications really need to be offered to treat these conditions. These medicines include Brahmi-Vati, Saraswatarishta, Brahmi (Bacopa monnieri), Shankhpushpi (Convolvulus pluricaulis), Vacha (Acorus calamus), Mandukparni (Centella asiatica), Abhrak-Bhasma, Trivang-Bhasma and Suvarna-Bhasma.

Many people affected with TS can lead a normal life with appropriate medications. Treatment needs to be tailor-made for each individual person. Psychiatric therapy might also work for several people affected with TS.

Natural medicine

Tics may be because of nutritional shortages, genetic conditions, Tourette syndrome, body immune system breakdown, allergies, or tension. Tension and stress and anxiety can increase the frequency of facial tics. Emotional trauma can trigger tics which can disappear when the psychological disorder is treated. Tics because of psychological trauma or stress can enhance or disappear with hypnotherapy, Emotional Liberty Technique (EFT), energetic treatment, Neuro-Linguistic Programs (NLP) yoga, Tai Chi, music therapy, homeopathy, Interactive Metronome, cognitive behavioral therapy, HEMI Sync, acupuncture, massage, and scalp acupuncture. Secondary mood disorders can get worse the intensity of tics.

Dealing with and recovery facial tics or Tourette's syndrome with normal amino acids is the basis for Orthomolecular Medicine. Big dosages of naturally found proteins called amino acids can repair the imbalance in the brain and fix its breakdown. These amino acids are inexpensive and are used in restorative dosages much bigger than those levels typically found in food. The concept of orthomolecular medicine is based upon using very large doses of vitamins, minerals, amino acids, or botanical extracts for the cellular repair work and enhancement of typical brain activities and motor activities.

Lithium mineral salt might help this client if there is Tourette's syndrome, but it would not help for a lot of other kinds of facial tics. Botanicals that may deal with tics and lower tics and convulsions include kava, skullcap, valerian, St John's Wort, peppermint, black cohosh, dragon bone, prunella, arose hips, Go Teng, Tian Men Dong, Bai Shao, Yin Chen Hao. Orthomolecular medicine uses consists of magnesium, zinc, calcium, B Vitamins, and chromium in addition to the botanicals to support recovery.

Orthomolecular medicine uses big restorative doses of carnitine, tryptophan, taurine, GABA, and 5-HTP. Theanine, GABA, and 5-HTP can work well for tics caused by tension. These amino acids should be used long- term for Tourette's syndrome and you might want to think about IV therapy in the absolute worst cases for at least 9 months.

This patient may have severe allergies and gain from the elimination of genetically modified foods. The diet must be altered to omit unsaturated fats, caffeine, nicotine, artificial sweeteners, food ingredients, food dyes, alcohol, and high fat meats. Try to eat free range chicken, natural meat, organic or in your area produced eggs, and limitation red meat to twice per week. You should always eat breakfast reasonably high in protein. This might consist of whey protein, almond milk, or soy protein. Walnuts, yogurt, almonds, pumpkin seeds, sunflower seeds, and pecans are great snack foods ideas. Remember that corn is often a genetically customized food. Popcorn can be a pretty good junk food if you are certain that it is not genetically modified. Organic or locally grown vegetables and fruits are the best health options. Avoid foods that are usually contaminated with pesticides or heavy metals. Plant fruit trees in your yard for more fresh fruit.

Brain-Based Treatments

The part of the brain associated with a lot of movement conditions is called the basal ganglia. The classic movement disorder associated with malfunction of the basal ganglia is Parkinson's Disease. Although Tourette's Syndrome and Parkinson's Illness are both related to issues in the basal ganglia, the fundamental problems in the basal ganglia are rather different in these two conditions.

For instance, in Parkinson's Disease, certain cells and areas of the basal ganglia degenerate and die off. Unlike Parkinson's Illness, the basal ganglia in kids with TS don't normally degenerate, but rather heads out of balance. This distinction, degeneration as occurs in Parkinson's Illness versus imbalance, which is more typical in TS, might clarify why, in general, clients with Parkinson's illnesses generally worsen with age and why most Tourette's symptoms get much better and minimize with time.

Some amazing research that has been just recently published suggests that part of the basal ganglia has spikes of extreme electrical activity in clients with Tourette's Syndrome. This excessive electrical activity in the brain produces the involuntary tics and twitches seen in Tourette's clients. The more conscious, upper part of the brain, works to suppress this abnormally increased activity in the lower parts of the brain at the basal ganglia. Researchers actually believe that this top down suppression of over activity might explain why the tics of Tourette's Syndrome generally take place when the kid is at rest and seldom are seen with conscious exercise. The scientists believe that this top down suppression of the over activity is the brain's way of compensating for and ultimately minimizing the symptoms of Tourette's Syndrome. So as the kid's brain ages, the brain can compensate for the irregular activity responsible for the tics of Tourette's Syndrome.

The question becomes what, if anything can be done to either

1. Straight suppress the irregular electrical hyperactivity in the basal ganglia that is related to the signs of Tourette's Syndrome or

2. Enhance the higher parts of the brain that compensate for the unusually elevated electrical activity and suppress it?

Different researchers have used either deep brain or vagal nerve stimulation to reset the electrical activity in the brain and to suppress the signs of Tourette's Syndrome in patients who couldn't react to any other type of treatment. Regrettably these brain stimulation techniques are intrusive and carry great threat. However other scientists in Germany showed that non-invasive brain stimulation may be possible through simple electrical stimulation of the vagus nerve on the external element of the ear.

This means that the irregular electrical activity in the brain that produces lots of the signs of Tourette's Syndrome may be reduced or modulated by a moderate external electrical stimulus delivered to the skin around the external ear. In addition, methods of chiropractic neurology may offer techniques that might boost the top down suppression of the irregular electrical spike activity. These strategies are essentially brain exercises that have the prospective to enhance the upper brain's natural ability to reduce the hyperactivity of the lower parts of the brain that are accountable for many of the signs of Tourette's syndrome.

Controlling It with Neurofeedback

A private with Tourette's syndrome might be sitting in the classroom, the boardroom, or out shopping in public when unrestrained cursing begins. This sudden eruption of language, which the person has no control over, is awkward to them and mortifying to people hearing the outburst. For this reason, some people with Tourette's will simply stay locked up at home, which then leads to other issues such as anxiety.

While the specific cause of Tourette's syndrome is still a secret, the majority of medical doctors and scientists really believe it relates to a breakdown of signals in the brain that manage concentration and emotion. As the criteria used for diagnosing this disease is so strict, the majority of people actually believe that Tourette's is an unusual condition, but in truth, this is a reasonably common disorder.

Because of the social inhibition that can result from dealing with Tourette's syndrome, and how Tourette's can result in so much anguish for the patient, an incredible amount of research has gone into treatments and therapies for the disorder. One treatment that has been getting a substantial amount of attention is neurofeedback therapy. Scientific studies show great possible for the efficiency of this interference, which trains the client to control brain wave frequencies, which in turn, may manage and even stop the symptoms.

Interestingly, it has been discovered through this thorough research that other conditions are typically related to Tourette's syndrome, consisting of attention deficit condition, depression, obsessive-compulsive condition, stress and anxiety, hypersexuality, and other highly addicting habits. This new information supplies even more reasons neurofeedback appears to be an extremely effective methods of stopping and controlling the various symptoms of Tourette's.

The tics of this disease typically react quickly and positively to neurofeedback. Another challenge is that with so many symptoms, Tourette's requires an extremely trained therapist that can figure out the suitable procedure for clients.

Therefore, therapists will recognize the most uncomfortable symptoms of Tourette's syndrome on a patient-by-patient basis and begin the neurofeedback training there first, and after that slowly carry on to resolve additional problems. Just because of this, addressing Tourette's syndrome with neurofeedback may need more diligence and time than some other conditions, but with a figured out client and a skilled therapist, the possibilities are exciting.

Remember, it is common for a Tourette's syndrome patient to stay on medication while going through neurofeedback therapy, as the individual begins to get symptoms under control, the level of pharmaceutical management would likely decrease. If you have this illness or know of somebody who does, it would be well worth talking to your mental health expert about the possibilities connected with neurofeedback. For a person with Tourette's syndrome, it could mean getting his or her life back without residing in fear of doing or saying something inappropriate.

How to Live with the Syndrome

It can be very hard to cope with Tourette's syndrome. Yes, it is a mental disability that is extremely tough to explain to others, even really loved ones. Yet, there are lots of people who deal with this condition and are attempting to live typical lives. It can be hard to do this, given that extremely few people know about the condition.

Here are several methods to cope with Tourette's syndrome:

1. Develop a positive mindset. Always believe that you will prosper. Thinking that things will fail will do extremely little to boast your self-esteem and give you a very good quality of life.

2. Can you remember success types success. It is essential to put yourself into effective circumstances as much as possible. The more successful you are now, the more successful you will be in the future.

3. Accept your impairment without judging yourself or feeling bad about it. People can be really oblivious and unjust. Make sure that you respect yourself as much as possible. Keep in mind there is nothing you can do about your special needs. So, try to accept it.

4. Be assertive and supporter for yourself as much as possible. Be an advocate for yourself. Don't be dependent on others. Do things yourself and take pride in what you have achieved, no matter how bit. Understand your rights. learn to be assertive to get what you really need.

5. Stay active. Workout can alleviate tension and help you feel better about yourself. It can also relieve tension and help control your condition, specifically in circumstances when your feel overwhelmed.

6. Know your strengths and weak points. Everybody, despite capability or impairment, has strengths and weaknesses. Know what yours are. Build on your strengths and find a way around your weaknesses.

7. Request aid, if you need it. Be specific when asking for aid. What is it precisely that you need? Take care and succinct with your demand, and you will make sure to ask happily.

By taking these steps, you will be living as well as you can with Tourette's syndrome. And you will have the ability to tell people what you need and others will quicker accept you as a result.

Six More Coping Tips

By following the 6 suggestions, you can best cope with the condition and even help other ones to understand you better.

1. Be a role model. There are numerous people with Tourette's syndrome. We should not presume that people will be judgmental of us. So, we have to act assertive and self-assured, even when we feel a bit afraid.

2. Don't welcome pity. The even worse thing that we can do is to welcome a pity party for what we are going through. Everyone has different hardships. So, it is necessary to cope and to prosper, regardless of the simple fact that you might have Tourette's syndrome.

3. Know who your true friends are. People who really love us truly and are real friends won't laugh at us or make fun at our disabilities. If you find that somebody is a lot like that towards you, have absolutely nothing to do with that person and find people who will really care about you for who you are.

4. When you get torn down, get up rapidly. We all get torn down. We can't do much about that. But we sure can do something about how we react to hurts from other ones. So, when somebody hurts you, carry on. Try and have absolutely nothing with do with the person or have a frank conversation with the person.

5. Choose your battles. Coping with Tourette's syndrome is hard enough. People will be ignorant of your condition and what you are going through. So, it is important not to strike everyone who says a wrong word that will harm us. Since we are delicate anyways, we need to pick our fights and make certain that we don't overreact to things that are little.

6. Offer people more than one chance to comprehend you. Since Tourette's syndrome is so little understood, we must give other individuals more than one chance to understand us. If they keep hurting us on purpose, though, it is time to carry on and connect with other people.

By taking these steps, you will be handling Tourette's syndrome in the best possible way, and you will be attempting your best to live in a world that very much doesn't comprehend what you are going through.

Despite the fact that medications can be helpful in minimizing tic intensity, the majority of people with TS will not need prescription medications for their tics. The requirement for medication depends on the seriousness of tic signs, the presence of co-occurring issues and the person's overall practical capability. For instance, those with extremely frequent tics, but who aren't distressed by them, might not want or require medication. On the other hand, some with less extreme signs may experience problems in social, school or work functioning and choose to chase after medication treatment. Ultimately, the choice about whether or not to begin a medication must take these realities into account. Despite the fact that not everybody might need medication for their tics, it is important for everybody to know what the treatment options are.

Prior to starting medication, it is necessary to find a certified clinician (e.g. doctors, nurse specialists and psychologists) for an examination. Although lots of clinicians can provide examination and treatment services, it is important to identify a clinician who has the expertise and the time to do the examination and be able to begin and keep track of medication treatment. The evaluation must at minimum determine issues related to tics and any co-occurring conditions. Other important components of a very good evaluation consist of the patient's general health, family history of any medical and psychiatric problems, treatment history including which medications the person is taking presently or may have taken in the past. A comprehensive assessment is a vital primary step for making good medication choices.

The next step is a discussion with the clinician about the actual results of the examination, the prepare for treatment and readily available treatment choices. This conversation ought to concentrate on the problems recognized and the reasons for selecting a specific treatment plan. Although people with tics tend to chase after treatment when signs are substantial, it is important not to be in way too much of a hurry. Some tic worsening may solve in time and for that reason may not require treatment with medication (e.g. tic increases as a result of enjoyment during holidays or vacations). It is worth the time it requires to make a very good choice about whether to begin taking medication.

The last step is the real treatment trial a process of finding the best dose with the fewest adverse effects. The majority of clinicians begin medication with a low dose and increase the dose in time so as to reduce tic severity while keeping medication side effects to a minimum. It is incredibly essential when starting medication to report both the advantages and negative effects to the clinician so that the best and safest dose of medication can be found.

Although everybody wants to take the lowest possible effective dose of medication, in some cases higher dosages may be needed and should not, in concept, be avoided or cause undue concern. Finding the best dose of medication for a kid can be more complex than for grownups. Although children often use lower doses than adults, father and mother should not automatically presume that children always require low doses of medication. Actually, kids sometimes need dosages comparable to those of adults or perhaps higher. It is a good idea to deal with clinicians experienced in treating children and who are actually aware of such distinctions and take them into account when prescribing medication. With the right clinician a medication trial can be accomplished-- even in children.

Since a lot of medications do disappoint advantage instantly, the pacing of dose changes is also important. Taking too long to increase the dose of a medication might unnecessarily extend suffering; increasing doses too rapidly may inadvertently overshoot the efficient dose and increase the threat of side effects. Once an optimum medication dose is determined, ongoing tracking is required to examine for continuing benefit, negative effects and adherence to the medication plan.

After a period of effective treatment, the clinician might suggest minimizing the dosage of medication in order to recognize the lowest dose that is required to preserve good tic control. As tic signs regularly wax and wane and improve gradually, regularly decreasing the dose of medication is a fundamental part of tic treatment. Practically all tic reducing medications should be reduced gradually to find the lowest reliable dosage.

A sluggish decrease in medication is particularly important for those who have been on tic suppressing medications for an extended time period. The same goes for stopping medication; the dosage ought to be minimized slowly and after that stopped, and never ever stopped quickly. Stopping tic suppressing medications abruptly can actually cause tics to get worse in a way that would not otherwise occur with a more steady decrease in dose. Some patients actually develop short-term motor motions called withdrawal dyskinesia from stopping medication too rapidly. Your clinician will recommend a safe step-by-step program for decreasing dosage till the medication is ceased completely.

Issues that co-occur with TS might also respond to medication. At the end of the assessment, it is not unusual for people with TS to become more knowledgeable about just how these co-occurring problems have been affecting their lives. If co-occurring problems are more hindering or stressful than the tics, clinicians may suggest that the co-occurring problems be treated first instead of dealing with the tics. For example, a kid with mild to moderate tics may have more significant problems with attention and concentration at school, or stress and anxiety and worries in the home. Dealing with these other issues initially may be useful in ways in which the child and family hadn't initially thought about. By addressing these issues first, operating at school and in the home might improve and make it less very likely that the tics will require treatment.

Those managing both tics and another co-occurring issue may require treatment for both conditions. Often attending to 2 (or more problems) might require a treatment strategy that includes two (or more) medications. While it is always most basic to use one medication, taking 2 medications to deal with 2 or more issues is routine practice, and should not trigger excessive concern. That said, while careful tracking and great communication are necessary when on a single medication, these preventative measures are seriously important when medication combinations are prescribed.

Some people with TS lead extremely hard lives. At times their difficulties are caused by their symptoms, sometimes by how others treat them, and in some cases their issues are because of the choices and choices they produce themselves. Although this pamphlet focuses on medication treatment, it is really crucial to note that not all the problems an individual with TS faces can be fixed by taking medication or lowering tic signs. Actually, mental treatments may be the most essential and important very first treatment step for tons of with TS.

The medications used for decreasing tic severity or treating co-occurring conditions come from different drug classes. Within each class there are certain medication options a clinician and patient may choose. That is why, people with TS and their families should talk about with their clinicians the particular symptoms to be targeted for medication treatment and the particular medication to be used. The following area is organized by class of medication and after that within each class are the particular medication choices.

There is no medication that has been found or developed specifically for the purpose of decreasing tic severity. Rather, medications developed to deal with other medical and psychiatric conditions have been later found to be helpful in minimizing tics. As a result, most of the published information about medications for tic reducing will refer to their use for other conditions without mentioning their usefulness in dealing with TS. The information below describes fundamental info about how these medications are frequently prescribed and how they are used in dealing with TS.

Antipsychotics are the most efficient group of medications for minimizing tic seriousness. They are categorized as significant tranquilizers or antipsychotic medications as they are typically prescribed for hallucinations, misconceptions and issues with thinking and organization in people with psychosis. These medications have also been classified as antiemetics because they can be effective in lowering serious queasiness and throwing up. There are certain medications thought about to be part of the antipsychotic class, and the majority of these have been tried in people with TS.

Antipsychotic medications are believed to be practical for TS symptoms just because of their ability to reduce dopamine function in the brain. Dopamine is a neurotransmitter-- a brain chemical-- which is involved in afferent neuron interacting with each other. Some antipsychotics have a lot of particular power to minimize dopamine working and some have less power. Antipsychotics also differ in their effect on other brain neurotransmitters (e.g. serotonin, Norepinephrine, acetylcholine). The influence of a particular antipsychotic on dopamine and other neurotransmitters will affect the medication's possible benefits as well as its side effects.

Antipsychotic medications with tested efficacy for lowering tic severity include the typical antipsychotics haloperidol (Haldol), pimozide (Orap), and the irregular antipsychotic risperidone

(Risperdal). Others antipsychotics might also be useful [e.g. fluphenazine (Prolixin)] even if they have not been particularly studied in TS. In general, antipsychotics with the best dopamine stopping activity are the most effective for minimizing tics. Nevertheless, the decision about which medication a person should take depends upon which medication might benefit the particular patient best. Clinicians may suggest using a medication besides one with a long performance history as stabilizing the advantage and side effects might fit the individual better than medications more frequently recommended.

Decreasing dopamine function is handy for minimizing tic intensity, but decreasing dopamine function might also result in undesirable results on motor control like tightness, slowed movements and unwanted contraction (i.e. dystonic responses, tremor and restlessness). These side effects are really common enough that people should be aware of them and comprehend the best way to manage them. They are all reversible either by decreasing the dosage or sometimes by terminating the medication. Additionally, some of these motor adverse effects can be managed by taking ant cholinergic medications like benztropine (Cogentin), diphenhydramine (Benadryl) and trihexyphenidyl (Artane). Anticholinergic medications may be started with an antipsychotic to stop the development of undesirable motor side effects, or given after motor side effects develop to decrease discomfort. Likewise, as antipsychotics are tranquilizers and decrease agitation for people with psychosis, they may be too tranquilizing for people with TS, leading to sedation or lowered cognitive efficiency.

In general, the dosage of antipsychotic used to deal with psychosis is significantly higher than dosages used for tic suppression. A dosage of antipsychotic for tic suppression may vary from 5-30% of the daily dose needed for psychosis. There are always exceptions to such general declarations, but usually, high doses of antipsychotics for tic suppression aren't more handy than lower dosages, cause more side effects and therefore aren't advised.

To improve the treatment for psychosis and to reduce the danger for motor negative effects, irregular antipsychotics were developed. Atypical antipsychotics have reasonably less influence on dopamine and more effect on other neurotransmitter systems. Just because of the lesser impacts on dopamine, irregular antipsychotics might be a better choice for people with TS who are sensitive to motor adverse effects triggered by the typical antipsychotics. In addition, irregular antipsychotics may impact other neurotransmitter systems too, resulting in a broader series of benefits (e.g. enhanced state of mind or impulse control) for people with TS. Although atypical antipsychotics might have less threat for motor adverse effects, some appear to increase cravings and trigger weight gain. Recently there has been increasing concern about antipsychotic-induced weight gain being connected with the development of metabolic issues including non-insulin dependent diabetes (i.e. type II diabetes) and raised cholesterol.

In addition to the common side effects of antipsychotics described above, it is important to know about 2 extremely unusual, but substantial issues of antipsychotic treatment-- tardive dyskinesia and antipsychotic malignant syndrome. Going over these problems of antipsychotic treatment in this pamphlet does not mean that they are likely to happen; rather they are defined here to put the threat of these negative effects into perspectives and allay issues of individuals who may be thinking about antipsychotic treatment.

Alpha Adrenergic Agonists
Another class of medications typically used for tic suppression are the Alpha Adrenergic Agonists coniine and guanfacine (Catapres and Tenex respectively). These medications are marketed to control hypertension, but have been prescribed for some other conditions, consisting of drug withdrawal syndromes and tics. Precisely how alpha adrenergic agonists minimize tic severity is not understood, but it might be associated with reduced central nervous system arousal.

Does of alpha agonists for tic signs are usually lower than those used in the treatment of hypertension. Since alpha agonists are brief acting, for optimum tic control multiple doses throughout the day (2-4 dosages) may be needed. Although some people with TS may have a relatively significant response to alpha agonists, many experience more modest advantage than what is normally observed when taking antipsychotic medications. On the other hand, the negative effects profile of the alpha agonists is milder than that of the anti-psychotics. The most common negative effects is sedation which can happen even at relatively low dosages. Some kids on alpha adrenergic medications have exhibited increased irritability.

Both clonidine and guanfacine can be found in a patch form. When connected to the skin, the spot launches the medication into the blood stream more gradually than tablets hence offering more convenient dosing and consistent medication results. The spot choice reduces the need for tablet taking several times each day, and may have less side effects than the pill form. Nevertheless, some people develop a skin rash at the site of the patch prompting discontinuation.

Guidance for Families

These three Tic Disorders are called based on the types of tics present (motor, vocal/phonic, or both) and by the length of time that the tics have been present. Below are the requirements that a medical professional or other health care expert will use to detect TS or other Tic Disorders.1 There is no test to confirm the diagnosis of Tic Conditions, but sometimes, tests might be required to eliminate other conditions.

Tourette Syndome (TS), also called Tourette's Disorder
1) A minimum of 2 motor tics and at least 1 vocal (phonic) tic have been present, not always at the same time.
2) Tics may wax and subside in frequency but have occurred for more than 1 year.
3) Tics started to appear right before the age of 18.

4) Tics aren't brought on by making use of a substance or other medical condition.

Consistent (Persistent) Motor or Vocal Tic Condition
Either motor tics OR singing tics have existed for more than 1 year; cannot be both motor and vocal tics.

Provisionary Tic Disorder
Motor and/or singing tics have existed for less than 1 year, and have not met the criteria for TS or relentless (persistent) motor or vocal tic disorder.

Other Crucial Things To Learn About Tics
They can change in type, strength, or place.
They often increase with stress, excitement, anxiety, and fatigue.
Some may be repressed, but only temporarily.
They might be minimized during focused activities.
They can be preceded by a premonitory urge, described as a sensory or mental experience that occurs before a tic.

Onset Of Tics And Period
Tics usually arise between the ages of 5 and 7 years, generally with a motor tic in the head or neck region. They tend to increase in frequency and severity between the ages of 8 and 12 years and can range from moderate to extreme. Many people with TS see enhancements by late teenage years, with some ending up being tic-free. A minority of people with TS continue to have persistent, severe tics into the adult years.

Tics happen in as lots of as 1 in 5 school-aged kids at some time, but may not persist.

TS and other Tic Conditions integrated are approximated to take place in more than 1 in 100 (1%) school-aged kids in the United States.

TS occurs in 1 in 160 (0.6%) school-aged kids. The reported frequency for those who have been identified with Tourette is lower than the true number, most likely as tics usually go unacknowledged. TS impact all races, racial groups and ages, but are 3-4 times more typical in boys than in girls.

There are no trustworthy occurrence estimates of TS and other Tic Disorders in adults. Nevertheless, they are expected to be much lower than in kids as tics tend to decrease into late teenage years.

Typical Co-Occurring Conditions
People with TS often have other psychological, behavioral, or developmental conditions that may be present prior to the beginning of tics. While tics are the main signs, these co-occurring conditions might trigger more problems and can be more irritating than the tics themselves.

Amongst people detected with TS, it is estimated that 86% have been detected with at least one of these additional conditions.

The most typical co-occurring conditions consist of the following:
Attention Deficit/Hyperactivity Disorder (ADHD): Issues with concentration, hyperactivity, and impulse control.

Obsessive Compulsive Disorder or Behaviors (OCD/OCB):
Recurring, undesirable invasive thoughts and/or repeated behaviors. These ideas result in obsessions, which are unwanted habits that the individual feels he/she must perform over and over or in a certain way.

Behavioral or Conduct Issues: Hostility, rage, oppositional defiance or socially improper behaviors.

Stress and anxiety: Extreme worries or fearfulness, including excessive shyness and separation anxiety.

Learning Disability: Reading, writing, mathematics, and/or info processing difficulties that aren't related to intelligence.

Social Abilities Deficits and Social Performance:
Trouble developing social skills; keeping social relationships with peers, members of the family, and other individuals; and acting in an age-appropriate manner.

Sensory Processing Issues: Strong sensory choice and sensitivities associated with sense of touch, noise, taste, smells, and movement that interfere throughout the day.

Sleep Disorders: Trouble falling or staying asleep.

Dealing with Ts And Other Tic Conditions.
Most often, tics are moderate, and treatment is not needed. Nevertheless, if tics are moderate to severe, they might really need direct treatment. If co-occurring conditions are present, it may be essential for your child or you to be evaluated and dealt with for the other conditions first or concurrently, as they can be more impairing than tics. In every case, it is necessary to be educated as a parent of a child or a specific with Tourette, in addition to inform people around your child or you (with his/her authorization).

Bullying Prevention.
The nature of TS signs and the lack of comprehending that they are uncontrolled behaviors make children with TS particularly susceptible to being bullied, which can contribute to solitude and stress and anxiety.

It is important to educate all relatives, instructors, good friends, and peers about TS. Be sure to involve your kid in the conversations. It can be valuable to emphasize that TS is a medical condition and that telling your child to stop ticking is not a technique (similar to telling somebody, you have blue eyes. Stop having blue eyes.) and is likely to trigger significant frustration.

Consider what circumstances make tics better and even worse. There are strategies your child can use to help manage tics in various circumstances. More information can be found in the Education area of the tool set.

In school settings, it can be really handy to educate instructors and peers by presenting to the class, or demonstrating the HBO documentary,
Academic Issues And Behaviors In School.
Demand direct input from your child's teachers about his/her scholastic performance and behavior in the classroom.

Think about instructional screening to assess co-occurring learning and attention difficulties.

Talk with your kid's school about 504 Strategies or Customized Education Programs (IEPs), which can greatly enhance the scholastic performance of students with tics.

Comprehensive Behavioral Intervention For Tics (Cbit).
Comprehensive Behavioral Intervention for Tics (CBIT, pronounced see-bit) is a behavioral, non-medicated treatment that has been shown in scientific studies to decrease tics in children and grownups. A study has also suggested CBIT to be as efficient as medication in most cases, and is usually recommended as the first treatment technique.

There are 3 main parts to CBIT:
1. Ending up being more aware of tics.
2. Developing contending reactions that are incompatible with the tics and less visible.
3. Making changes in daily activities that can be useful in decreasing tics.

Extra screening might be needed for co-occurring conditions that would obstruct of CBIT, just like neglected ADHD or considerable Oppositional Bold Condition (ODD). Determine whether certain therapies are practical from a logistical perspectives. Is there an experienced CBIT supplier readily available locally? Is there transportation? Does your insurance cover these services? Only therapists who have received specific training in CBIT should provide this treatment.

Prospective Impact On Education.
Tourette Syndrome (TS) is hard for some teachers to comprehend as every student has different symptoms, which can change, wax, and wane. Some instructors may not be well informed about methods and techniques for recognizing the requirements of students with TS, or the most reliable teaching approach. Besides the tics, lots of common co-occurring

conditions can be impairing, just like Attention Deficit/Hyperactivity Disorder (ADHD), handwriting problems, sensory incorporation or sensory processing disorders, obsessive-compulsive habits, and social skills deficits.

Acknowledging the Check In School Settings
Educators and families should know indications that may point to underlying symptoms of the common conditions that co-occur with TS. It is essential to acknowledge the indications so that the extra support in school can be provided for students with Tourette Syndrome or other Tic Disorders. The following are very common indicators that extra assistance might be required:

Difficulty going to or staying at school
A collaborative and positive working relationship with the school can help in a sincere conversation to determine why this may be occurring and then developing a proactive/positive plan to help.

Conduct problems in the house or school
Concentrating on when, where, and why behaviors are occurring will reduce the chance of making presumptions and penalizing the child. The Tourette Association provides several resources tailored toward attending to difficult behaviors at school and strategies for these troubles.

Considerable hesitation to finishing work in school and/or homework
This could be a sign that the child has problems in the following parts: handwriting problems, problems with memory, processing delays, or difficulties with company. It might also be due to fatigue, which can increase tics and signs of other disorders and make focusing more difficult. A conference with proper school staff (such as the instructor, counselor, or other ones dealing with your child) to talk about why this is happening can be useful. A preliminary assessment or re-evaluation may be necessary to identify if particular abilities deficits are the reason for this.

Dropping grades
It prevails for students with tics and co-occurring conditions to receive great grades in primary school and then experience a decrease in the grades in middle and high school. An upgraded education evaluation/assessment will assist in figuring out if hidden signs might be accountable and assist in determining appropriate assistances.

Boost in tics, stress and anxiety, and obsessive compulsive behaviors
This may be a sign that a meeting with school staff is needed to discuss any changes that might be increasing stress and anxiety. Conversations should consist of problems with peers and particular instructors or support workers.

Difficulty socializing with peers
Screen for social language deficits, as they are very common troubles for students with TS that can severely affect peer interactions and friendships. Using

social stories might not work since students with TS often know what to do and say, but are inconsistently able to perform as they know they should and are in some cases capable of doing.

Loss of interest in favored activities
Consider the environment to figure out if there is something or somebody
increasing stress and anxiety. It might also be because of some obsessive-compulsive behaviors related to efforts to achieve perfection.